Praise for Dr. Yang, Jwing-Ming ...

"His depth of knowledge and his superb teaching style make him among the most valuable members of this community."

— Pat Rice
Director, *A Taste of China*

"Having used martial arts on the street for real, I am skeptical of many of today's 'famous masters'—there are many who write and talk but who cannot truly do. After meeting Dr. Yang in person and observing his skill, I came away impressed that he is indeed one who can do as well as write."

— Captain John P. Painter, Ph.D.
Publisher *IAM Magazine*,
American Rangers Law Enforcement   Martial
Training Institute

"Dr. Yang has surely made a valuable contribution to the community by making Chinese material about ancient Chinese weapons accessible for western readers interested in the martial arts."

— Christian Weinert
in *Journal of Asian Martial Arts*

"Dr. Yang has an enormous amount of knowledge of Western science and Chinese cultural skills. He is famous throughout the Qigong and martial arts world. Anybody who seriously studies martial arts or Qigong has heard his name, seen his articles, or read his books. For many years he has worked hard to promote Chinese martial arts and Qigong and brought his vast knowledge and experience of traditional Chinese skills to the West."

— Michael Tse
Publisher, *Qi Magazine*

NORTHERN SHAOLIN SWORD

NORTHERN SHAOLIN SWORD

SWORD

DR. YANG, JWING-MING
AND
JEFFERY A. BOLT

YMAA Publication Center
Boston, Mass. USA

YMAA Publication Center
Main Office:
    4354 Washington Street
    Boston, Massachusetts, 02131
    617-323-7215 • ymaa@aol.com • www.ymaa.com

10 9 8 7 6 5 4 3 2 1

Copyright ©2000 by Yang, Jwing-Ming
All rights reserved including the right of reproduction in whole or in part in any form.

ISBN:1-886969-85-X

Edited by James O'Leary
Cover design by Richard Rossiter

Publisher's Cataloging in Publication

(Prepared by Quality Books Inc.)

Yang, Jwing-Ming, 1946-
    Northern Shaolin Sword : form, techniques &
applications / by Yang Jwing-Ming and Jeff Bolt.
— 2nd ed.
        p. cm — (Martial arts-external)
        Includes index.
        LCCN: 00-101608
        ISBN: 1-886969-85-X

        1. Swordplay—China. 2. Martial arts.
        I. Bolt, Jeffrey A., 1956- II. Title.

GV1147.Y26 2000   796.8'6
                            QBI00-517

Disclaimer:
The authors and publisher of this material are NOT RESPONSIBLE in any manner whatsoever for any injury which may occur through reading or following the instructions in this manual.
The activities, physical or otherwise, described in this material may be too strenuous or dangerous for some people, and the reader(s) should consult a physician before engaging in them.

Printed in Canada

To Grandmaster Li, Mao-Ching

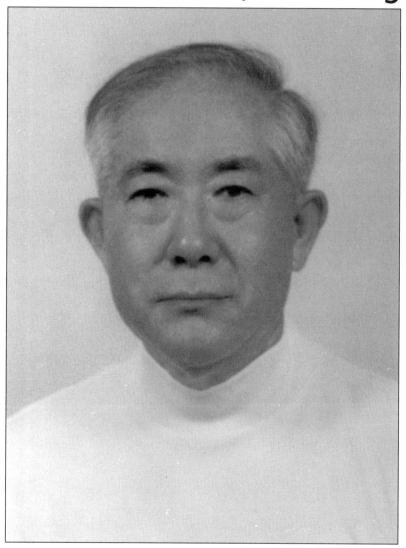

Romanization of Chinese Words

This book uses the Pinyin romanization system of Chinese to English. Pinyin is standard in the People's Republic of China, and in several world organizations, including the United Nations. Pinyin, which was introduced in China in the 1950's, replaces the Wade-Giles and Yale systems. In some cases, the more popular spelling of a word may be used for clarity.

Some common conversions:

Pinyin	Also Spelled As	Pronunciation
Qi	Chi	chē
Qigong	Chi Kung	chē kǔng
Qin Na	Chin Na	chǐn nǎ
Jin	Jing	jǐn
Gongfu	Kung Fu	gŏng foo
Taijiquan	Tai Chi Chuan	tī jē chǔen

For more information, please refer to *The People's Republic of China: Administrative Atlas, The Reform of the Chinese Written Language,* or a contemporary manual of style.

Contents

About the Authors

Dr. Yang, Jwing-Ming, Ph.D. 楊俊敏博士

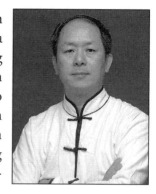

Dr. Yang, Jwing-Ming was born on August 11, 1946, in Xinzhu Xian (新竹縣), Taiwan (台灣), Republic of China (中華民國). He started his Wushu (武術) (Gongfu or Kung Fu, 功夫) training at the age of fifteen under the Shaolin White Crane (Bai He, 少林白鶴) Master Cheng, Gin-Gsao (曾金灶). Master Cheng originally learned Taizuquan (太祖拳) from his grandfather when he was a child. When Master Cheng was fifteen years old, he started learning White Crane from Master Jin, Shao-Feng (金紹峰), and followed him for twenty-three years until Master Jin's death.

In thirteen years of study (1961-1974) under Master Cheng, Dr. Yang became an expert in the White Crane Style of Chinese martial arts, which includes both the use of barehands and of various weapons such as saber, staff, spear, trident, two short rods, and many other weapons. With the same master he also studied White Crane Qigong (氣功), Qin Na (or Chin Na, 擒拿), Tui Na (推拿) and Dian Xue massages (點穴按摩), and herbal treatment.

At the age of sixteen, Dr. Yang began the study of Yang Style Taijiquan (楊氏太極拳) under Master Kao Tao (高濤). After learning from Master Kao, Dr. Yang continued his study and research of Taijiquan with several masters and senior practitioners such as Master Li, Mao-Ching (李茂清) and Mr. Wilson Chen (陳威伸) in Taipei (台北). Master Li learned his Taijiquan from the well-known Master Han, Ching-Tang (韓慶堂), and Mr. Chen learned his Taijiquan from Master Zhang, Xiang-San (張祥三). Dr. Yang has mastered the Taiji barehand sequence, pushing hands, the two-man fighting sequence, Taiji sword, Taiji saber, and Taiji Qigong.

When Dr. Yang was eighteen years old he entered Tamkang University (淡江大學) in Taipei Xian to study Physics. In college he began the study of traditional Shaolin Long Fist (Changquan or Chang Chuan, 少林長拳) with Master Li, Mao-Ching at the Tamkang College Guoshu Club (淡江國術社) (1964-1968), and eventually became an assistant instructor under Master Li. In 1971 he completed his M.S. degree in Physics at the National Taiwan University (台灣大學), and then served in the Chinese Air Force from 1971 to 1972. In the service, Dr. Yang taught Physics at the Junior Academy of the Chinese Air Force (空軍幼校) while also teaching Wushu. After being honorably discharged in 1972, he returned to Tamkang College to teach Physics and resumed study under Master Li, Mao-Ching. From Master Li, Dr. Yang learned Northern Style Wushu, which includes both barehand (especially kicking) techniques and numerous weapons.

In 1974, Dr. Yang came to the United States to study Mechanical Engineering at Purdue University. At the request of a few students, Dr. Yang began to teach Gongfu (Kung Fu), which resulted in the foundation of the Purdue University Chinese Kung Fu Research Club in the spring of 1975. While at Purdue, Dr. Yang also taught college-credited courses in Taijiquan. In May of 1978 he was awarded a Ph.D. in Mechanical Engineering by Purdue.

In 1980, Dr. Yang moved to Houston to work for Texas Instruments. While in Houston he founded Yang's Shaolin Kung Fu Academy, which was eventually taken over by his disciple Mr. Jeffery Bolt after he moved to Boston in 1982. Dr. Yang founded Yang's Martial Arts Academy (YMAA) in Boston on October 1, 1982.

In January of 1984 he gave up his engineering career to devote more time to research, writing, and teaching. In March of 1986 he purchased property in the Jamaica Plain area of Boston to be used as the headquarters of the new organization, Yang's Martial Arts Association. The organization has continued to expand, and, as of July 1, 1989, YMAA has become just one division of Yang's Oriental Arts Association, Inc. (YOAA, Inc.).

In summary, Dr. Yang has been involved in Chinese Wushu since 1961. During this time, he has spent thirteen years learning Shaolin White Crane (Bai He), Shaolin Long Fist (Changquan), and Taijiquan. Dr. Yang has more than thirty-one years of instructional experience: seven years in Taiwan, five years at Purdue University, two years in Houston, Texas, and seventeen years in Boston, Massachusetts.

In addition, Dr. Yang has also been invited to offer seminars around the world to share his knowledge of Chinese martial arts and Qigong. The countries he has visited include Argentina, Barbados, Belgium, Bermuda, Botswana, Canada, Chile, England, France, Germany, Holland, Hungary, Ireland, Italy, Latvia, Mexico, Poland, Portugal, Saudi Arabia, South Africa, Spain, Switzerland, and Venezuela.

Since 1986, YMAA has become an international organization, which currently includes sixty-one schools located in Argentina, Belgium, Canada, Chile, France, Holland, Hungary, Ireland, Italy, Poland, Portugal, South Africa, the United Kingdom, the United States, and Venezuela. Many of Dr. Yang's books and videotapes have been translated into languages such as French, Italian, Spanish, Polish, Czech, Bulgarian, Dutch, Russian, and Hungarian.

Dr. Yang has published twenty-six other volumes on the martial arts and Qigong:

1. *Shaolin Chin Na;* Unique Publications, Inc., 1980.
2. *Shaolin Long Fist Kung Fu;* Unique Publications, Inc., 1981.
3. *Yang Style Tai Chi Chuan;* Unique Publications, Inc., 1981.

4. *Introduction to Ancient Chinese Weapons;* Unique Publications, Inc., 1985.

5. *Qigong for Health and Martial Arts;* YMAA Publication Center, 1985.

6. *Northern Shaolin Sword;* YMAA Publication Center, 1985.

7. *Tai Chi Theory and Martial Power;* YMAA Publication Center, 1986.

8. *Tai Chi Chuan Martial Applications,* YMAA Publication Center, 1986.

9. *Analysis of Shaolin Chin Na;* YMAA Publication Center, 1987.

10. *Eight Simple Qigong Exercises for Health;* YMAA Publication Center, 1988.

11. *The Root of Chinese Qigong—The Secrets of Qigong Training;* YMAA Publication Center, 1989.

12. *Muscle/Tendon Changing and Marrow/Brain Washing Chi Kung—The Secret of Youth;* YMAA Publication Center, 1989.

13. *Hsing Yi Chuan—Theory and Applications;* YMAA Publication Center, 1990.

14. *The Essence of Taiji Qigong—Health and Martial Arts;* YMAA Publication Center, 1990.

15. *Qigong for Arthritis;* YMAA Publication Center, 1991.

16. *Chinese Qigong Massage—General Massage;* YMAA Publication Center, 1992.

17. *How to Defend Yourself;* YMAA Publication Center, 1992.

18. *Baguazhang—Emei Baguazhang;* YMAA Publication Center, 1994.

19. *Comprehensive Applications of Shaolin Chin Na—The Practical Defense of Chinese Seizing Arts;* YMAA Publication Center, 1995.

20. *Taiji Chin Na—The Seizing Art of Taijiquan;* YMAA Publication Center, 1995.

21. *The Essence of Shaolin White Crane;* YMAA Publication Center, 1996.

22. *Back Pain—Chinese Qigong for Healing and Prevention;* YMAA Publication Center, 1997.

23. *Ancient Chinese Weapons;* YMAA Publication Center, 1999.

24. *Taijiquan, Classical Yang Style;* YMAA Publication Center, 1999.

25. *Tai Chi Secrets of Ancient Masters;* YMAA Publication Center, 1999.

26. *Taiji Sword, Classical Yang Style;* YMAA Publication Center, 1999.

Dr. Yang has also published the following videotapes:

1. *Yang Style Tai Chi Chuan and Its Applications;* YMAA Publication Center, 1984.

2. *Shaolin Long Fist Kung Fu—Lien Bu Chuan and Its Applications;* YMAA Publication Center, 1985.

3. *Shaolin Long Fist Kung Fu—Gung Li Chuan and Its Applications;* YMAA Publication Center, 1986.

4. *Shaolin Chin Na;* YMAA Publication Center, 1987.

5. *Wai Dan Chi Kung, Vol. 1—The Eight Pieces of Brocade;* YMAA Publication Center, 1987.

6. *The Essence of Tai Chi Chi Kung;* YMAA Publication Center, 1990.

7. *Qigong for Arthritis;* YMAA Publication Center, 1991.

8. *Qigong Massage—Self Massage;* YMAA Publication Center, 1992.

9. *Qigong Massage—With a Partner;* YMAA Publication Center, 1992.

10. *Defend Yourself 1—Unarmed Attack;* YMAA Publication Center, 1992.

11. *Defend Yourself 2—Knife Attack;* YMAA Publication Center, 1992.

12. *Comprehensive Applications of Shaolin Chin Na 1;* YMAA Publication Center, 1995.

13. *Comprehensive Applications of Shaolin Chin Na 2;* YMAA Publication Center, 1995.

14. *Shaolin Long Fist Kung Fu—Yi Lu Mai Fu & Er Lu Mai Fu;* YMAA Publication Center, 1995.

15. *Shaolin Long Fist Kung Fu—Shi Zi Tang;* YMAA Publication Center, 1995.

16. *Taiji Chin Na;* YMAA Publication Center, 1995.

17. *Emei Baguazhang—1; Basic Training, Qigong, Eight Palms, and Applications; YMAA* Publication Center, 1995.

18. *Emei Baguazhang—2; Swimming Body Baguazhang and Its Applications;* YMAA Publication Center, 1995.

19. *Emei Baguazhang—3;* Bagua Deer Hook Sword and Its Applications YMAA Publication Center, 1995.

20. *Xingyiquan—12 Animal Patterns and Their Applications,* YMAA Publication Center, 1995.

21. Simplified Tai Chi Chuan—Simplified 24 Postures & Standard 48 Postures; YMAA Publication Center, 1995.

22. Tai Chi Chuan & Applications—Simplified 24 Postures with Applications & Standard 48 Postures; YMAA Publication Center, 1995.

23. *White Crane Hard Qigong;* YMAA Publication Center, 1997.

24. *White Crane Soft Qigong;* YMAA Publication Center, 1997.

25. *Xiao Hu Yan—Intermediate Level Long Fist Sequence;* YMAA Publication Center, 1997.

26. *Back Pain—Chinese Qigong for Healing and Prevention;* YMAA Publication Center, 1997.

27. *Scientific Foundation of Chinese Qigong;* YMAA Publication Center, 1997.

28. *Taijiquan, Classical Yang Style;* YMAA Publication Center, 1999.

29. *Taiji Sword, Classical Yang Style;* YMAA Publication Center, 1999.

About the Authors

Mr. Jeffery A. Bolt

Jeff Bolt was born in Cincinnati, Ohio, in 1956. In 1975, while pursuing an engineering degree at Purdue University in Indiana, he joined the Purdue Chinese Kung Fu Research Club to study under Dr. Yang, Jwing-Ming. It was during the next 4 years that Jeff studied Northern Long Fist and Southern White Crane Gong Fu as well as Taijiquan from Dr. Yang. He went on to become an instructor in Gong Fu as well as Taijiquan.

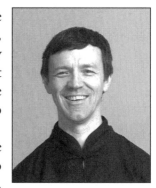

In December of 1978, Jeff graduated with a Bachelor of Science in Engineering and moved to Houston, Texas. From 1980 to 1982, Dr. Yang was also employed as an engineer in Houston, giving Jeff the opportunity to continue advanced training with him.

When Dr. Yang moved to Boston in 1982, Jeff continued teaching at the school that Dr. Yang founded and continues to teach there to this day. Shortly after Dr. Yang's departure from Houston, Jeff had helped Dr. Yang with the original issue of *Northern Shaolin Sword* and became co-author of that book. Jeff is also the co-author of *Shaolin Long Fist Kung Fu* published by Unique Publications.

Over the next four years, Jeff became active in various open martial arts tournaments, eventually hosting this country's first all Chinese martial arts competition to be held on a national level. This was in the fall of 1986. In 1987, *Inside Kung Fu Magazine* inducted Jeff into its Hall of Fame for Outstanding Martial Arts Promotions.

Since 1986, the number of Chinese martial arts events in the country continue to increase from year to year. Jeff went on to host several more national level Chinese martial arts events in Houston and hosted three events in Orlando, Florida. His third event in 1997 included a national Pay-Per-View event and featured what many have considered the most exciting Chinese martial arts demonstrations they have ever seen in this country. It also featured several Chinese Sanshou fighting matches for the first time on national Pay-Per-View TV.

In 1991, Jeff helped to create the United States Chinese Martial Arts Council. The council's goal was to further organize the Chinese martial arts in the United States. A few years later, the Council merged with another organization to become the USA Wushu Kungfu Federation. The USAWKF continues to promote and organize Chinese martial arts through regional and national competitions. Jeff has served as the Vice President of that organization since it's inception.

Since 1986, Jeff has attended and either judged others or helped to administer many Chinese martial arts events around the country. He also continues to teach Chinese martial arts at his school in Houston, Texas all while continuing a full-time engineering career.

Foreword

by Sam Masich

"The art of swordsmanship is extremely elusive and subtle; its principles are most secret and profound. The Dao has its gate and door, its Yin and Yang... You should resemble a modest woman and strike like a ferocious tiger... Your opponent endeavors to pursue your form and chase your shadow, yet your image hovers between existence and non-existence." These were the words Yue Ne (越女), an unparalleled swordsman of The Yue Kingdoms (越國) in the late Spring and Autumn Period (Chun Qiu, 722-484 B.C., 春秋), when asked by her King how he could strengthen his army.

More than any other weapon, the straight sword is associated with spiritual refinement as much as with martial efficacy. In ancient Chinese culture the sword was a symbol, not only of law and legacy, but of cutting through illusion and attachment to ego. While the way of the blade will never again reign supreme in an age of technological weaponry, it retains a place deep in our psyche's imaginings of honor, courage, and discipline. From this place we may find that when we pick up the straight sword, we hold, not an obsolete piece of metal and wood, but a tool which can connect us directly with the balance point between the extremes of Yin and Yang in our own nature. There are few examples today of English language books which present traditional Chinese straight sword practices. Three important routines are detailed in this generous volume, each of which provides a solid foundation for external and internal style martial arts sword study. By re-releasing this improved edition, Dr. Yang, Jwing-Ming and Jeff Bolt, have continued to make an invaluable contribution, not only by providing an excellent reference guide for learning, but by preserving and encouraging the survival of an important key to the understanding of Chinese physical culture. I sincerely hope that aspirants will mine this source thoroughly with an intention toward extending themselves both as martial artists and as the bearers of a unique approach to self cultivation.

Sam Masich
June 30, 2000

Preface—First Edition

by Dr. Yang, Jwing-Ming

The Jian (劍), a narrow-blade, double-edged sword, has been respected as the "King of Short Weapons" in China for millennia. This is so both because wielding requires the highest of skill, and because the sword user must strive to the heights of spirit and morality. In addition to the obvious self-defense uses, swords were commonly carried by scholars for their elegance. Also, because of its beauty, the Jian has always been popular for use in dance.

Although the art of the sword has enjoyed a glorious past, its future is uncertain. Modern culture leads people away from its study for several reasons. First, the gun replaced the sword as a personal weapon a century ago because of its ease of operation and greater killing potential. This leads people to believe that sword techniques have no practical value. Second, there are few masters qualified to teach, and thereby to preserve, the artistry of handling the sword. Finally, proficiency in sword techniques requires much time, patience, and practice, and few people today seem willing to exert the energy necessary to learn the ancient art of the Chinese sword.

The study and practice of sword techniques, however, like that of any martial art, has value far beyond that derived from merely perfecting the technique. First, it has intrinsic historical value. This art form has been developing for over 4,000 years and represents a great development of human culture. Second, there is the more conventional aesthetic value. The human body in motion in the martial arts, like the natural movement of animals, displays a sense of native growth and completion. Like a fine dancer, the accomplished martial artist exhibits total control of his or her body. Third, it promotes good health. Like any sport, perfecting the art of the sword requires extensive physical training, which results in a strong, finely tuned body. Fourth, sword technique retains its personal defense value because it trains one's perceptions and reactions, allowing for quick and correct response to any situation. Finally, the most important aspect of the art of the sword remains its moral value. The practitioner must learn patience, perseverance, and humility. If the student persists and concentrates, sword art will strengthen his spiritual confidence and power.

This book will present an introduction to Northern Shaolin Long Fist Jian (sword) techniques, and the practical applications of these techniques. Chapter One will cover general information about the Jian, including basic knowledge, history, structure, and the spirit or soul of the sword way. Chapter Two will present fundamental training and the principles of sword techniques, which build the foundation of practical application. Chapter Three will introduce a fundamental sword sequence, the "San Cai Jian" (三才劍) and its applications. This sequence is the only one known in which the techniques in the sequence match themselves, so that it can be done as a two person set. Chapter Four presents another well known and more advanced sword sequence, the "Kun Wu Jian" (崑峿劍). The application of every technique is included. Chapter Five contains the famous and very long Qi (戚) family's sequence "Qi Men Jian" (戚門劍), which demonstrates advanced sword skills and brings the student to a higher level of sword application. Naturally, the application of each technique is given. In order to practice and master the sword techniques for real situations, practice with a partner is practically a necessity. Therefore, Chapter Six will present two person fighting forms. After the fundamental uses and the two person matching practice has been understood and mastered, training in free sparring can then be started. The authors hope that this book will provide practicing martial artists with an interest in the sword with a more comprehensive understanding. They also hope this book will encourage people to study, practice, research and compete in this elegant and beautiful art.

Dr. Yang, Jwing-Ming

Preface—New Edition

by Dr. Yang, Jwing-Ming

Since I resigned from my engineering job in 1984, and placed all my effort into presenting the Chinese martial arts and Qigong culture to the West, I have had the chance to travel and offer seminars in more than 20 countries. In addition, the YMAA organization has expanded rapidly from only a couple of schools ten years ago, to the current forty-eight schools spread through fourteen countries.

From these years of teaching around the world, I have learned that one of the most difficult areas of knowledge and skill to pass down to students is the art of the narrow blade sword. The most difficult part of this process is conveying the essential feeling of the art. Generally speaking, learning the external forms (i.e., movements) of the art may take only a few days or weeks. However, it will take many years of continuous pondering and practice to reach the deep feeling of the art. It is hard for a student to commit to this effort in today's society. It is difficult to teach a student any discipline that is linked to spiritual cultivation. Normally, the appearance or the look of the art can be limited, but its internal quality is unlimited. In Chinese martial society, it is said: "One hundred days of fist (i.e., barehand), one thousand days of spear, and ten thousand days of sword."* This implies that the starting point for training is a proficiency in the skills and basic foundation of the barehand techniques. This requires a continuous and cumulative effort of consecutive practice sessions focused on basic skill development (i.e., one hundred days). This, however, is the easy part. Once the barehand techniques are assimilated, it will take "one thousand days" to do the same for the spear, and ten thousand days for the sword. Then you are ready to really enjoy and master the elegant art of the sword.

It is because of this demanding training that sword work has traditionally been considered the highest expression of skill in Chinese martial arts. It includes the training of not just the external skills and movements, but also the internal cultivation of Qigong. From the external into the internal, the emotional origin of the techniques into calm and graceful action requires wisdom and a spiritually cultivated mind. From sword training, you learn how to challenge yourself constantly, and to master yourself. From this process of self-conquest, you glean clues into the meaning of life.

I have been attracted by sword techniques since I started martial arts, when I was fifteen years old. The principles of southern sword, and its manner of use, are very different from those of the northern sword. Nevertheless, since they all build upon the same basic root and theory, once you have learned one, it becomes much easier to pick up the other. I have been more fortunate than many others, since I have had

---

* 百日拳，千日槍，萬日劍。

a chance to learn both the southern sword (White Crane) and northern sword (Long Fist). This has provided me with a broader scope of understanding, both in skills and theory.

Still, learning and practicing sword are difficult. Interest in this art is also increasing. I believe that this is because contemporary attitudes have changed from more material enjoyment to favoring spiritual cultivation. I believe that the twenty-first century for all humanity will focus on self-cultivation. Therefore, it is more important than ever to introduce those profound spiritual arts that have been passed down to us from the past. Only by learning from the past correctly and continuing to develop this knowledge, will we be able to carefully preserve the arts.

I hope this new edition will serve this purpose. I also hope the readers will treat the learning process as a life time project instead of temporary attraction. Only if you have this commitment and attitude, are you able to reach the profound level of the art.

Dr. Yang, Jwing-Ming

Preface—New Edition

by Mr. Jeffery A. Bolt

I don't claim to be an expert by any means in the use of the Chinese straight sword. However, over the many years that I have practiced with this weapon, I have learned that to master it takes a complete devotion of time and discipline. It is intricate, graceful, artistic, and extremely effective.

I have noticed over the many years that I have attended Chinese martial arts competitions that relatively speaking, the straight sword competitors in the traditional kung fu divisions were few and far between. Still, the quickness and spirit as well as complexity of this weapon have indeed been promoted, however, in the modern wushu events. It is no wonder that the Chinese have chosen to include this event as one of its anchor programs. The history of the sword is too vast and the beauty of it is too great to let it go by the wayside. I would guess that if it weren't for the structured wushu programs promoted by the Chinese wushu institutes, we would see much less of this weapon than we do today.

While many skills of the straight sword are indeed demonstrated by competition hopefuls, in my opinion it is still extremely rare that these competitors could ever be able to actually use this weapon effectively or even properly in real application. But then, there is little reason to spend so much time in today's age to practice this weapon or any martial arts weapon for actual combat.

It could then only be for the sake of discipline, tradition and/or pure personal interest that one would practice the straight sword to its highest level. For those who are interested, this book serves as an introduction to the history, techniques and application of this weapon. I hope that this book will spark the interest of the readers to seek further information as well as instruction for learning the Chinese straight sword, and to research this weapon and preserve this treasure of our art.

Jeff Bolt

Acknowledgments

Thanks to John Gilbert Jones and Russell Steinberg for general help with the work. Thanks to the editors, Michael Braun and James O'Leary, and special thanks to Alan Dougall and Erik Elsemans for proofing the manuscript and contributing many valuable suggestions and discussions. Thanks also to John Casagrande, Jr. for the drawings.

CHAPTER 1

Introduction

介紹

1-1. GENERAL INFORMATION

Many martial artists who have studied Chinese martial arts for quite a few years may still have many questions about the structure, use, history, geographical background, etc., of the sword (Jian, 劍). This is because most students of Chinese martial arts have not also studied Chinese culture. Very little of the available martial literature has been translated into European languages, and the number of qualified and knowledgeable masters is steadily diminishing. This section will discuss general information about the Jian history, structure, and the sword spirit will be discussed in sections 1-2, 1-3, and 1-4 respectively.

Definition of the Sword. There are two kinds of weapons commonly called a sword by the Western world. One is the double-edged, narrow-blade weapon that is called a "Jian" (劍) in Chinese. The other is the single-edged weapon with a wide blade, which in China is called a "Dao" (刀), and will be referred to here as a saber. If either a double or single edged weapon is shorter than the forearm, it is called a dagger (Bi Shou, 比首). These can be easily hidden in one's boot or sleeve. This volume will present the techniques for using the northern style sword only; saber and dagger techniques will be covered in a later volume.

Names of Swords. Chinese swords were most often named. The names usually designated either the sword's origin or the sword's owner. The origin could be the name of the mountain where the ore used to make the sword was found (e.g., Kun Wu Jian, 崑崙劍), the place where the sword was forged (e.g., Long Quan Jian, 龍泉劍), or the smith who forged the sword (e.g., Gan Jiang and Mo Xie, 干將，莫邪). Of course the sword could be named by its owner as he pleased (e.g., Judge Li's sword "Rain Dragon"). In addition the sword could be named for the style of the sequence in which it was designed to be used (e.g., Taiji Jian, 太極劍).

Names of Sword Sequences. Sword sequences are commonly named for a mountain near where the sequence was created such as Wu Dan Jian (武當劍), for a division or style of Gongfu, such as Taiji Jian (太極劍), or for the person who composed the sequence such as Qi Men Jian (戚門劍). It can also be named by the creator of the sequence as he pleases (e.g., San Cai Jian, 三才劍).

Functions of the Sword. More than most weapons, the sword serves a variety of purposes. First, the sword has always been used as a defensive rather than an offensive battle weapon. Because it is shorter than the spear, the halberd, or many of the other large battle weapons, it lacks their long-range killing potential. In battle the sword was mainly carried for use when the soldier's main weapon was lost or broken. Second, in peace time the sword was treated as a defensive weapon and was carried by scholars and magistrates as well as by soldiers. Third, it showed the bearer's status. This function of the sword developed to the point that some swords carried by scholars (Wen Jian, 文劍) were so ornate that they could not easily be used for fighting, although this was unusual before the advent of the gun. Fourth, the sword was an integral part of many dances.

Why the Sword is Respected. Sword art has been respected in China not only because the techniques and skills needed are hard to learn, but more importantly because the morality and spirit of the practitioner have to be of a very high order in order to reach the highest level of the art. The training is long and arduous, and most people first learn to use other short weapons such as the saber in order to build a foundation.

Carrying the Sword. In China the sword was either slung from a belt around the waist (Figure 1-1) or was strapped to the back with shoulder straps (Figure 1-2). The way a person carried his sword depended on the weight and length of the sword—double swords and martial swords (Wu Jian, 武劍) were ordinarily carried on the back—as well as on personal preference.

How to Inspect a Sword. There are two occasions for inspecting swords: by the swordsman after using the sword, and by an admirer of the weapon. There are several conventions to be observed when one inspects a sword. First, the sword is always passed from person to person by handing it hilt first. This minimizes the danger of accidental injury. Second, the sword handler never touches the blade with bare skin because the oils and salt from the skin will result in corrosion. Third, the blade is always kept at least eight inches (20-30 cm.) away from the nose and mouth, since moisture from the breath can also result in corrosion on the blade. Fourth, the sword handler never points the sword at another person, both for safety and from courtesy. Fifth, the edge of the blade is inspected by holding the sword by its hilt in one hand and resting the other end against the scabbard (Figure 1-3). If there is no scabbard, use the thumbnail of your free hand (Figure 1-4) or your sleeve (Figure 1-5), so that, again, the blade is protected from corrosion.

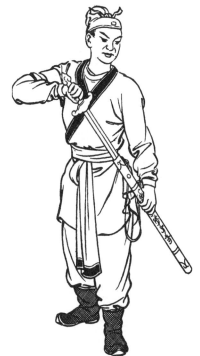

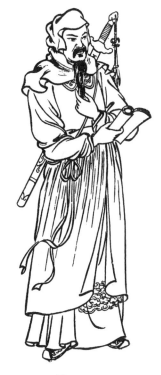

Figure 1-1

Figure 1-2

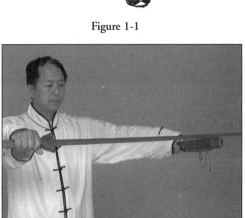

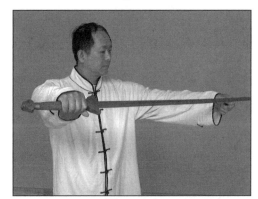

Figure 1-3

Figure 1-4

How to Select a Sword. Because of the success of modern metallurgical techniques, there is no need for a student to make his own sword as was sometimes done in ancient times. Excellent swords can be bought at most martial arts supply stores. A modern Jian of spring steel is the equal or superior to any common sword of antiquity. Plated, untempered swords are also available and are considerably cheaper than the spring steel ones; however, these are definitely practice swords. Selection criteria for a Northern Style sword are as follows:

1. It should be 30 inches long, or longer, and the hand guard should point toward the sword tip rather than toward the hand.

2. The taper of the blade from hilt to tip should be smooth and steady, with no abrupt changes of width or thickness.

3. The blade must be straight when viewed down the edge (Figure 1-6).

4. The blade must be firmly mounted in the handle. It should not rattle when you shake it.

5. Spring steel blades must be flexible enough to bend 30 degrees and not retain any bow. The dealer may not like this test, so you must be firm about it.

6. The sword should balance at a point one third of its length from the hilt end (Figure 1-7). If it does not, the balance must be altered or it will not handle properly.

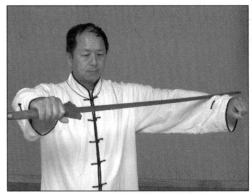

Figure 1-5

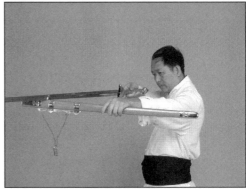

Figure 1-6

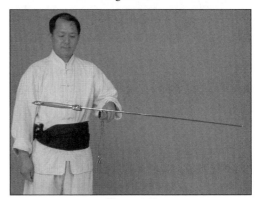

Figure 1-7

Sheathing the Sword. Formerly sword and scabbard were created as one interlocking assembly. Many of these units were spring loaded so that the sword leaped from the sheath when the latch was released. Even when not spring loaded, swords will frequently latch to the scabbard to insure their protection, and these latching scabbards have a stud at the open end. If you have such a sword, put it away by resting the hilt end of the blade on the stud, drawing the blade out to the tip, and letting the blade slide easily into the sheath. If the scabbard does not have this stud, the thumbnail must serve in its place. The first step in sheathing the sword is to place the thumb over the open end of the sheath so that it is half covered (Figure 1-8), and then to bring the sword around to rest the part of

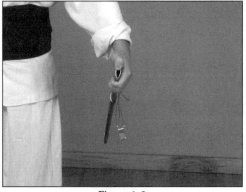

Figure 1-8

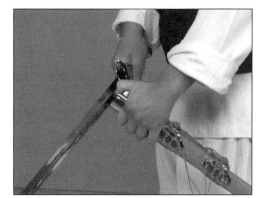

Figure 1-9

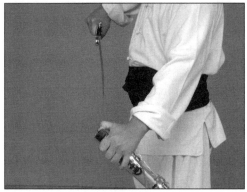

Figure 1-10

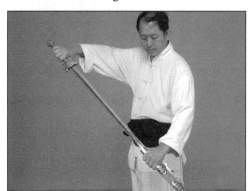

Figure 1-11

the blade closest to the hilt on the thumb and sheath (Figure 1-9). The second step is to slide the sword out to the tip so that the tip falls into the end of the sheath (Figure 1-10), remove the thumb, and slide the sword into the sheath (Figure 1-11). Practice carefully until sheathing the sword becomes natural.

Care of the Sword. In order to protect the sword from damage the following procedures must be observed:

1. When you show your sword to someone who knows nothing about it, be sure to tell the person what to do before giving it to him. This will protect your sword, and will also prevent anyone's getting cut.

2. Never lay the sword on the ground. It will absorb moisture from the ground, and in addition it might get stepped upon.

3. Never touch the blade with your bare skin. The sweat on your skin will cause the blade to corrode.

4. Avoid unnecessary cutting with the sword, since this will dull the blade and shorten the sword's life.

5. Always keep the sword sheathed when it is not in use.

6. After using the sword apply a light coat of grease to the blade.

7. Until your level of skill warrants it, don't use a real sword to practice. This will protect you as well as the sword.

Sword Proverbs. There is an old saying that "The staff is the root of all the long weapons, and the saber is the prerequisite for the short weapons," which implies that the long rod and the saber serve as a foundation for further work within each group of weapons. In Chinese martial society it is said that "The spear is the king of the long weapons, whereas the sword is the leader of the short weapons."[1] This saying implies that the spear and the sword are the hardest to learn of their kind, and that once someone can skillfully apply them in battle, he could take advantage of the techniques and skills required by the weapons and become the king and leader of the battle. There is also the previously mentioned proverb, "A hundred days of barehand, a thousand days of spear, and ten thousand days of sword."[2] From this proverb, one learns that the sword is the hardest weapon of all to learn. The reason for this is that the sword is light and requires more than ten years of internal power training to master the techniques for blocking heavy weapons. Also, because the sword is double-edged, more skill is required to use both edges effectively without dulling them. Therefore, it is said, "Sword uses speed and technique; saber requires cunning, trickery, and power." It is also said: "Saber, power, won by strength. Sword, soft, won by technique."[3] Finally, it is said, "The saber is like a fierce tiger, the sword is like a flying phoenix, and the spear is like a swift dragon."[4]

1-2. HISTORICAL SURVEY

The ancient Chinese regarded the sword as a very important weapon, as evidenced by the relatively large number of documents about it and the frequency with which swords turn up in archeological digs. It is the only weapon that has been used and admired continuously from the beginning of Chinese history to the present day.

Over time the sword has changed from a short, wide copper weapon to a long, slim steel one because of gradual improvements in metallurgy over thousands of years, and the techniques for using the sword have changed with these changes in qualities. The short, wide copper blade would not hold an edge and was soft, so that it could only be used at short range to hack and stab. Bronze is brittle, as is cast iron, therefore blades made of these materials would break easily when they were used for blocking. The longer the sword the longer the effective fighting range, so that the full array of fundamental techniques in use today were only made possible with the discovery of hardened and tempered steel in this millennium. The number of fundamental techniques has increased significantly from a very few with the early short, wide swords, to more than thirty in use today.

In examining the illustrations accompanying this chapter, the reader will see that swords differed from one dynasty to another, in shape, handle style and sheath decoration. The changes came not only because of developments in metallurgy, but also because of the influence of other cultures, particularly those of the invaders of China: the Mongolians, Manchurians, Tibetans, and Himalayans. China has in turn been a major influence on the cultures of nearby regions such as Korea, Japan, and Indo-China. For example, the Japanese Katana is similar in design to a sword used in China during the Tang Dynasty.

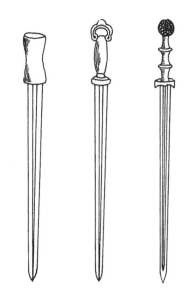

Figure 1-12. Sword styles of Zhou Dynasty.

The Chinese of 3000 to 4000 B.C., like other prehistoric societies, probably used the sticks and stones that lay about them to settle their disputes. Not until the time of the first recorded emperor, Huang Di (2690-2590 B.C., 黄帝), called the "Yellow Emperor" because he ruled the territory near the Yellow River, does evidence exist for weapons made of something other than stone. Huang Di had swords made of jade, copper, and gold. This period, therefore, marks the beginning of the metallurgical science in arms manufacturing in China.

Knowledge of Huang Di's weapons comes from discoveries near Zhuo Lu (涿鹿) of knives and swords, remnants of ancient battles between the emperor's forces and those of Chi You (蚩尤).

By the time of the Shang Dynasty (1751-1111 B.C., 商朝) swords made of copper alloys were in use. Bronze ushered in this era, but by its close, iron was being used.

The Zhou Dynasty (1111-221 B.C., (周朝) replaced the Shang following fierce warfare. Both emperors demanded better swords and in this way stimulated advances in metallurgy, with emphasis on finding alloys for stronger swords (Figures 1-12 and 1-13). As the power of the Zhou Dynasty diminished over time, the emperor's con-

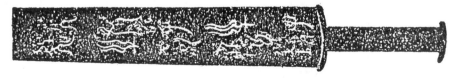

Figure 1-13. Engraved bronze sword (Zhou Dynasty).

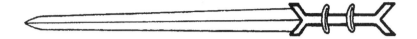

Figure 1-14. Typical sword style of Spring and Autumn Period.

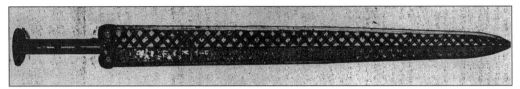

Figure 1-15. Cast copper sword of Gou Jian, King of Yue, discovered in 1965 (Warring States Period).

trol weakened, and China was thrust into a series of civil wars. This time is known as the Spring and Autumn Period (Chun Qiu; 770-403 B.C., 春秋) and the Warring States Period (Zhan Guo; 403-221 B.C., 戰國) (Figures 1-14 to 1-17). Each of the many warring factions strove to produce stronger and sharper weapons than before, and swordmakers of the day were held in the highest regard. Three of the most famous swordmakers of that period were Ou Ye Zi (歐冶子), Gan Jiang (干將), and Mo Xie (莫邪).

Ou Ye Zi forged two very famous swords, Ju Jue (巨厥) and Zhan Lu (湛盧). It is said that these swords were so sharp that if they were dipped in water, they would be withdrawn perfectly dry. Also famed are Gan Jiang and Mo Xie, who were husband and wife, and forged two swords that bear their names.

At the close of the Zhou Dynasty, the emperor Qin Shi (秦始) took power, establishing the Qin Dynasty (Figures 1-18 and 1-19) which lasted only fifteen years (221-206 B.C.). Qin Shi heard that the Wu Emperor He Lu (闔閭) had collected tens of thousands of swords from all over China, and had them buried with him when he died. Three hundred years later Emperor Qin Shi ordered his men to find these swords. After many years of searching and digging, the emperor had only a large hole for his efforts. Eventually the pit filled with water and came to be known as the Sword Pond (Figure 1-20) in Suzhou (蘇州).

During the Han Dynasty (206 B.C.-221 A.D., 漢朝) the process of alloying iron instead of copper was first described in the book *Huai Nan Wan Hua Shu (Huai Nan's Thousand Crafts,* 淮南萬華術), a book on metallurgy.

The Three Kingdoms Period followed (San Guo; 220-280 A.D., 三國) (Figures 1-21 and 1-22). The famous Cao-Cao (曹操) is reputed to have had swords that could cut iron as if it were mud. There is a story about his rival, Liu Bei (劉備) (Figure 1-23), that illustrates the effect of tempered iron swords. Liu, as a descendant of the Han imperial family, felt he had the duty to reunite China. To do this he occupied Shu (蜀) in western China (Sichuan Province, 四川省), and began preparing his

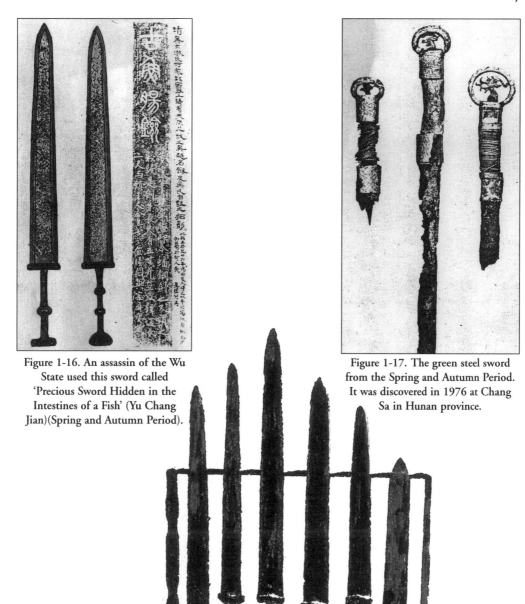

Figure 1-16. An assassin of the Wu State used this sword called 'Precious Sword Hidden in the Intestines of a Fish' (Yu Chang Jian)(Spring and Autumn Period).

Figure 1-17. The green steel sword from the Spring and Autumn Period. It was discovered in 1976 at Chang Sa in Hunan province.

Figure 1-18. Typical sword styles of Qin and Han Dynasties.

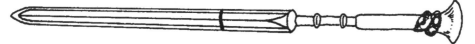

Figure 1-19. Copper sword with hilt shaped like a dragon's head (Qin Dynasty).

army for war. To recruit the best fighters, he often held and presided over contests, and one day two fighters stepped forward, one with an iron rod, the other with a saber. During the fight the rod wielder knocked the saber man down and brought his rod down to finish the fight. Everyone present was amazed when the iron rod broke in two as the saber blocked it. The maker of that saber, Pu Yuan (浦原) was found and immediately ordered to forge weapons for Liu Bei.

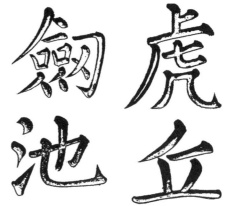

Figure 1-20. Stone carving at 'Sword Pond' in Suzhou.

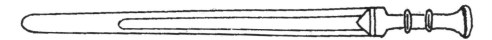

Figure 1-21. Drawing of two-foot long sword (Han Dynasty).

Figure 1-22. Copper sword (Han Dynasty).

From the Three Kingdoms Period until the Northern Zhou Dynasty (Bei Zhou; 557-581 A.D., 北周) (Figure 1-24) little is known about the weapons used, although copper is considered the predominant metal during this period.

The Sui and Tang Dynasties (581-907 A.D., 隋、唐) are the brightest and most peaceful eras in Chinese history. More famous scholars, poets, and other artists flourished, while the arts of war were neglected.

In 907 A.D. the country was once again divided into five parts known as the Five Dynasties (Wu Dai; 907-960 A.D., 五代), and then was reunited in the Song

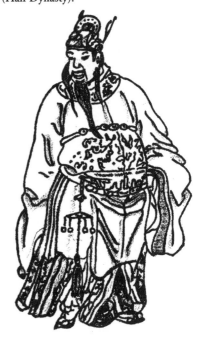

Figure 1-23. Emperor Liu Bei, ruler of Shu State during Three Kingdoms Period.

Dynasty (960-1280 A.D., 宋朝) (Figure 1-25). The Song ended with the invasion of Mongols (the Jin race, 金) who rounded the Yuan Dynasty (1206-1368 A.D., 元朝). This mixing of cultures resulted in more changes of sword styles (Figure 1-26).

In 1368 the Mongols were defeated by the Chinese and the Ming Dynasty (1368-1644 A.D., 明朝) began. Then the Manchurians invaded and formed the Qing Dynasty (1644-1911 A.D., 清朝). During these later dynasties steel and other alloys were used to make swords, which were longer than ever (Figures 1-27 to 1-29). There were three places during the Qing Dynasty famous for the quality of their weapons. Two are in Zhejiang Province (浙江省) in eastern China, Long Quan (龍泉) and Wu Kang (武康). The other is Qin Yang (沁陽) in Henan Province (河南省), the site of the Shaolin Temple (少林寺). This site attracted great swordmakers because of the quality of its water. No one is sure why the water is superior, but great arms have been forged in Long Quan for centuries because of it.

In the eighteenth century guns were introduced into China, and further development of the sword as a martial weapon ceased. Consequently the swords and other weapons used for martial arts study remain in the style of the Ming and Qing Dynasties.

1-3. SWORD STRUCTURE

The sword consists of two parts: the blade and the hilt or handle. Both edges of the narrow blade sword are sharp and the handle and sword body are always straight. The hand guard is always flat and parallel to the blade, rather than being circular or oval. Usually the sword is one continuous piece of metal and the hand guard and handle are slipped onto the butt end and held in place with a knob-shaped nut or with a pin or rivet. The blade or sword body is sharpened on both edges and the tip is either rounded or sharply pointed as described below. Swords are from 20 inches to 40 inches long and under 1.5 inches in width. The length is divided into three zones: the tip third, which is kept razor sharp and very

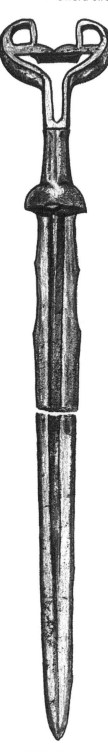

Figure 1-24. Copper sword (Northern Zhou Dynasty).

11

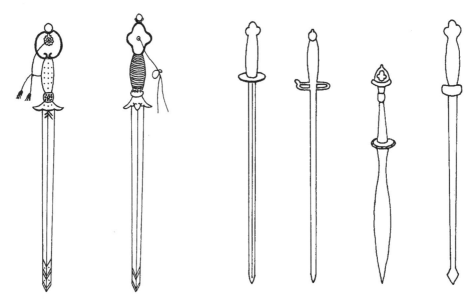

Figure 1-25. Sword styles of Song Dynasty.

Figure 1-26. Swords from Yuan Dynasty.

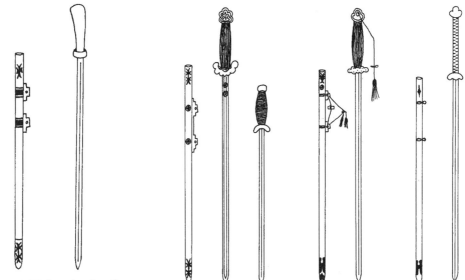

Figure 1-27. Sword styles of
Ming and Qing Dynasties.

Figure 1-28. Typical swords of Qing Dynasty.

flexible, the middle third, which is less sharp and stiffer, and the butt third which is
dull and very stiff, and is used for blocking. The sharp upper part can stab or cut to
kill the enemy. The duller lower part is used to slide or block the opponent's weapon.
The forward-pointing hand guard is used to lock an opponent's blade.

Types of Swords. Although there are numerous kinds of swords known, we will
only describe five here (Figure 1-30). Among these the first two (A and B) are the

most common swords, and are the kinds most often used today for practice. The other three kinds are specialized modifications of the first two. Although they can be used through most of the common sword techniques, there are additional special techniques made possible by their designs.

- Wen Jian (文劍) (Scholar's Sword): This sword is also called a female sword. It is long and light with a rounded tip. It is not commonly used for war, but for personal self-defense and for dancing. It was also commonly carried by scholars to present an elegant appearance, or was hung on a wall to decorate a room.

- Wu Jian (武劍) (Martial Sword): This sword, also known as a male sword, is long and heavy and has a pointed tip (because of its killing potential) and is mainly used in battle.

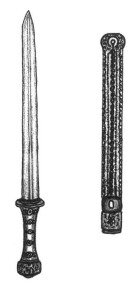

Figure 1-29. Sword used by Himalayan tribesmen (Qing Dynasty).

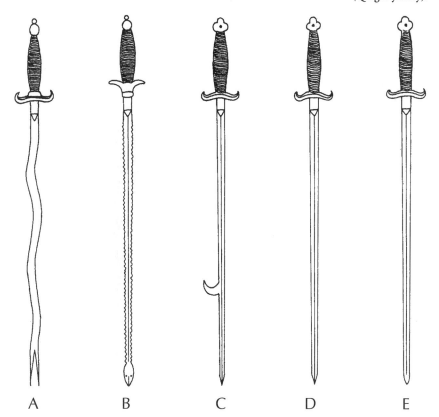

A   B   C   D   E

Figure 1-30. General types of swords.

- Wu Gou Jian (吳鈞劍) (Wu Hooked Sword): This sword was invented during the Wu Dynasty (222-280 A.D.), and is designed for cutting enemies' limbs or their horses' legs after blocking their weapons.
- Ju Chi Jian (鋸齒劍) (Saw-Toothed Sword): This sword has a serrated edge to give it greater cutting ability. The edge design probably originated when someone found that a badly knicked blade seemed to cut more viciously. The two holes in the tip of the sword resemble the eyes of a snake and make a whooshing noise when the sword is swung.
- She-She Jian (蛇舌劍) (Snake Tongue Sword): This sword has a wavy blade, which leaves a unique cutting ability. The double point may have given the fighter a way to catch his opponent's weapon at long range.

The Blood Groove. When a sword fighter stabs his enemy, the blade is fixed in the enemy's body by a vacuum, which makes it difficult to free the weapon. To solve this problem, most martial swords (Wu Jian, 武劍) were forged with a groove down each side of the blade called a blood groove. In battle one is faced with a multitude of enemies, so the warrior must be able to keep the blade free as much as possible in order to be able to defend himself. In street weapons the blood groove was less common, because they served a different purpose. Without the blood groove, freeing the imbedded sword requires that the swordsman either widen the wound by twisting the blade, or thrust the sword completely through the body to break the suction. The techniques later in this book include slashing motions designed to handle this problem.

The Tassel. Many swords in use today have a tassel hanging from the hilt to enhance their appearance. This tassel has no martial usefulness for the Jian, and it will not be included in the sequences in this book.

Historically, the scholar's sword, the dancing sword, and the decorative sword usually had a tassel, and the martial sword almost never did. The reasons for not using a tassel are: first, the tassel changes the balance of the sword, making it harder to handle; second, it can become entangled in the sword arm and in avoiding this the sword fighter's attention is distracted from the enemy; third, the opponent can grab the tassel and gain control of the sword.

The Sheath. There are two types of scabbard: the scholar sheath and the martial sheath. The scholar sheath is made of wood covered with snake or alligator skin to make it waterproof to protect the sword from moisture. The martial sheath is made of metal to enable it to withstand more abuse, and in addition the metal sheath can be used for blocking. Sheaths should be straight and stiff, and the brackets for the hanger must be tight and not slide up and down the sheath.

Sword Structure and Technique in Relation to Geography. The swords used today are almost all based on Qing Dynasty designs, so only these kinds of swords will be described here.

Northern Chinese tend to be taller than the southerners, and there are cultural differences as well, which resulted in north/south distinctions in both the structure and techniques of the sword.

Northern characteristics were as follows:

1. Swords are relatively long and narrow (the narrow blade reduces the weight). The average sword is six inches longer than arm length.

2. Sword guards face forward so the swordsman can lock the opponent's weapon.

3. Northern styles are more offensive or attack-oriented and specialize in long and middle range fighting.

Southern characteristics on the other hand were:

1. Swords are short, averaging arm length, and are relatively wide and thick (to increase the weight).

2. Sword guards slant backward toward the hilt to slide the opponent's weapon away to prepare for attack at close range.

3. Southern fighting styles are more defensive, specializing in short and middle range fighting.

1-4. The Sword Way

In ancient China the way of the sword was widely respected. This was so not just because its techniques and skills were hard to learn. The main reason was that moral and spiritual qualities were required in order to attain the highest artistic achievement. In order to build a proper foundation for the study of the sword, the martial artist had to master other short weapons, which meant that he had to spend a long time in preparation. Therefore the sword master (known in China as a "Jian Ke, 劍客) had to have willpower, endurance, and perseverance in order to get through the long and hard years of training.

Because the sword is mainly a defensive weapon, it requires a strategy of calmness in action, and to achieve this quality one needs patience, calmness, and bravery. Sword users commonly practiced meditation to acquire the calmness they needed. In addition to these qualities needed to develop the required level of skill, sword students learned additional virtues from their masters. The masters would try to develop these traits in their students by example, and by telling inspiring stories from history. First they taught loyalty. The student was taught to be loyal to his country, his master, his parents, and his friends. True loyalty even requires a willingness to die when necessary. The second trait learned was respect, which is closely related to humility. When one is humble one can then respect the style, other martial artists, parents, and the master. Another quality cultivated by the masters, and perhaps the most important, was righteousness. The student should act only in the interest of righteousness and justice.

Having achieved these traits the sword master was respected by the populace and would live an honored life.

References

1. 槍為長兵之王，劍為短兵之首。

2. 百日拳，千日槍，萬日劍。

3. 刀猛贏之以力，劍軟勝之以技。

4. 刀如猛虎，劍似飛鳳，槍比游龍。

CHAPTER 2

Fundamental Training and Practice

基本訓練與練習

2-1. INTRODUCTION

As was mentioned in Chapter One, the Jian is the king of the short weapons. Skill in the use of the Jian is built on a foundation of skill with the saber, which is called the root of the short weapons. Any martial artist who wants to master the Jian should first master the saber, otherwise it will be extremely difficult to understand the applications of the techniques and the source of the power in sword practice.

Although the saber is the root of the short weapons, its techniques and power applications are very different from those of the sword. For example, the saber uses muscle power. The blunt edge of the saber is designed for blocking vigorously, but this action cannot be done with the Jian. Since the sword is double-edged, using either edge to block will dull the blade. With the sword only the third of the blade nearest the hilt is designed for vigorous blocking. The sharpened part of the blade should not be allowed to contact the opponent's weapon. Therefore, a defensive attack without blocking is the best sword technique, and a sliding block followed by an attack is the second best. The least desirable defense is to block using the blunt area of the blade.

The fighting strategy is also different between saber and sword. The saber fighter will try to keep the enemy in the short and middle range in order to take advantage of the saber's vigorous blocking and attacking power. To do this the saber fighter always uses two hands together. One hand holds the saber while the other is used for coordination and balance or to grasp the enemy's wrist, arm, or weapon. The Jian fighter, however, tries to keep the enemy in the middle or long range in order to be able to use the razor sharp tip of the sword effectively. In addition, by keeping some distance from the opponent it is easier to avoid violent attacks.

For applying power the saber relies on muscle power, while the Jian uses muscle and internal power (Qi) together in order to defend against a heavy weapon or a strong attack. Because of the more refined power needed, the sword needs more technique, more skill, and more training time.

Even though there are so many differences between the saber and the sword, the saber is still the foundation of sword practice. It builds up the stances, dodging, and the basic forward and backward movements. It also builds the muscles required for sword practice. Most important of all, practicing the saber will help the student to understand in general the application and the fighting strategy of short weapons.

In learning the sword, the student should first cultivate the virtues of patience and calmness, and develop a firm will. He should understand the form and application of every movement.

To help the beginner to build up a good foundation of sword technique the second section of this chapter will introduce the key of balancing sword power. Fundamental stances will be discussed in section three. Power training for the sword will be in section four. Section five explains the key techniques of Northern Shaolin Long Fist sword, and finally, some fundamental practice forms and drills will be introduced in section six.

2-2. Grips and the Secret Sword

Mastering the sword requires learning to project power into the weapon, but if a person generated power only on one side of the body, disorders would result. To avoid this, sword practitioners hold the empty hand with the index and middle fingers extended and the thumb folded over the other two fingers (Figure 2-1). When power is extended into the sword, it is also projected from the extended fingers of the empty hand to balance the energy. This is known as the secret sword. It is also used for applying cavity press when appropriate. There is also an open hand secret sword (Figure 2-2), which is occasionally used in some styles, primarily those in which muscular strength dominates the sword application.

There are two basic ways to hold the sword: left-handed and right-handed. The left-handed grip (Figure 2-3) is used at the beginning of sequences, for defensive blocks, and to hold the sword while the right hand is used for a cavity press. The right-handed grip (Figure 2-4) is the usual grip for using the sword. The correct tightness must be maintained. If the grip is too tight you will lose flexibility and inhibit energy flow. If the grip is too loose, it is easy to be disarmed. The sword should be held like an egg, neither broken nor dropped. The grip should be alive.

2-3. Fundamental Stances

There are eight fundamental stances in Shaolin Long Fist Sword. The student should become proficient in every one. Each style of Gongfu has its own characteristic stances, and there are variations. Only Northern Shaolin Long Fist stances will be discussed here. It is important to understand that the basic stances are the foun-

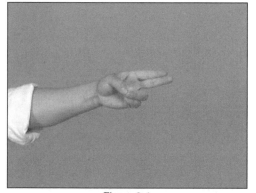

Figure 2-1

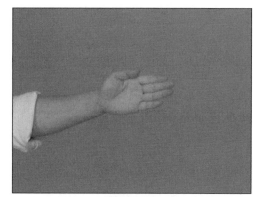

Figure 2-2

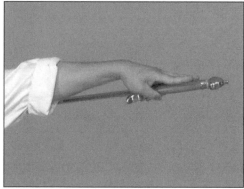

Figure 2-3

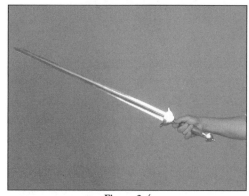

Figure 2-4

dation of the techniques. If the foundation is not firm, then the techniques cannot be performed properly, for they will be unstable. It is the leg forms that are important in the illustrations; the hand forms can vary for the same stance.

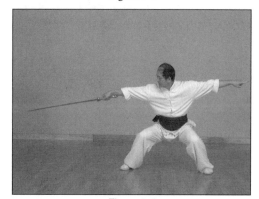

Figure 2-5

The Horse Stance (Ma Bu, 馬步). This stance (Figure 2-5) is the most fundamental and is especially valuable in building up the strength of the knees. To assume this stance, place the feet parallel slightly beyond shoulder width. Bend the knees until a 90 degree angle is formed between the back part of the calf and the thigh, keeping the back straight. It is important to concentrate on directing the power of the legs straight down and not to the side, as if standing on stilts. The knees should not bow out, but should be turned slightly inward. To practice this stance the student should begin by standing straight with both feet together and jump into the horse

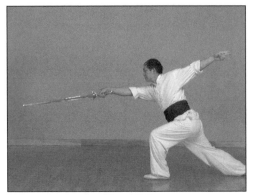

Figure 2-6

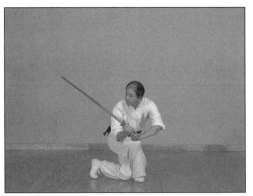

Figure 2-7

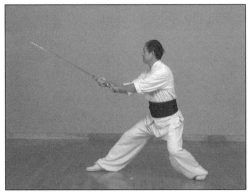

Figure 2-8

stance. The beginning student should try to maintain the stance for at least five minutes but no longer than ten.

The Mountain Climbing Stance or Bow and Arrow Stance (Deng Shan Bu, Gong Jian Bu, 蹬山步、弓箭步**).** This stance (Figure 2-6) is one of the most commonly used offensive stances. About 60 percent of the weight is on the front leg and 40 percent on the rear. The front knee is above the toes and the back leg is straight. The front foot should be turned inward about 15 degrees and the hips should face the direction of the forward leg.

The Crossed Leg Stance (Zuo Pan Bu, 坐盤步**).** This stance (Figure 2-7) can be used either for attack or defense. To assume this stance first stand in the Horse Stance. Raise the right toe while pivoting on the right heel. At the same time, turn right until the body is facing to the rear. During the turn the left foot pivots and turns on its toe. Bend the knees until the left knee is about one inch off the ground. In this final position the right foot is flat and the left is on its toes. For turning to the left reverse directions and weighting.

The Four-Six Stance (Si Liu Bu, 四六步**).** This is one of the most versatile stances in Wushu (武術) (Figure 2-8). From this stance, the martial artist can switch into various techniques with relative ease. In this stance, 40 percent of the weight is on the front leg, while 60 percent is on the back leg. The knee of the front leg should be turned slightly inward and bent. Never straighten the knee in this stance, because if a kick were to land on the stiffened knee, it could easily break it. The front foot should be at a 15 degree angle inward. In addition, the back knee must be flexed and turned inward toward the groin.

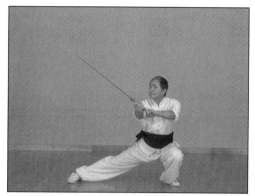

Figure 2-9

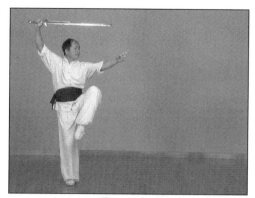

Figure 2-10

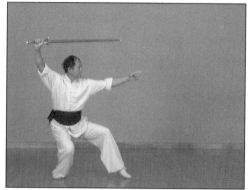

Figure 2-11

To change into the Four-Six Stance from the Horse Stance, turn the body to either direction so that the back leg holds 60 percent of the total weight and the front has 40 percent of the weight.

The Taming the Tiger Stance (Fu Hu Bu, 伏虎步**).** This stance (Figure 2-9) is generally used as a defense against high attacks. This stance has a particularly interesting origin. During the Song Dynasty (960-1280 A.D., 宋朝) a famous hero named Wu Song (武松) was suddenly attacked in the jungle by a huge tiger. As the tiger leapt at him, Wu Song drew his only weapon, a small dagger, and bent low to avoid the leaping tiger. While the tiger was hurling over him, Wu Song stabbed the tiger in the belly and killed it, thus taming the tiger.

To assume this stance, begin by standing in the Horse Stance. Squat down on the left leg until your thigh is parallel to the ground. The right leg should be extended straight out to the side. Both feet must be planted flat and the back is kept straight. Repeat on the right leg.

The Golden Rooster Stands on One Leg Stance (Jin Ji Du Li, 金雞獨立**).** This stance (Figure 2-10) is generally used to set up for quick leg attacks. To assume this stance raise one leg until the knee is as high as possible.

The False Stance (Xuan Ji Bu, Xu Bu, 玄機步、虛步**).** This stance (Figure 2-11) can be used for quick kicking. To assume this stance, place all the body's weight on one leg and lightly touch the ground with the toe of the other. To change legs, turn the body 180 degrees while shifting the weight from the rear foot to the front foot, which becomes the rear foot. Make sure the lead leg has no weight on it.

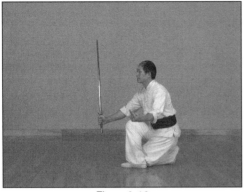

Figure 2-12

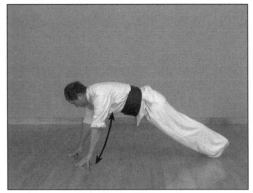

Figure 2-13

The Unicorn Stance (Qi Lin Bu, 麒麟步 **).** This stance (Figure 2-12) is another extremely versatile stance; the martial artist can easily move backward while having the ability to kick from the rear leg. The name of the stance comes from the belief that a unicorn had to bend its knee in order to bow. To assume the stance, start in the Horse Stance. Next, place the right leg behind the left leg. The knee of the right leg should be one inch above the ground and behind the left ankle. The right leg is on its toes and is at a 90 degree angle to the left foot. The left leg has about 80 percent of the weight. This stance is commonly used for withdrawal. Reverse this process for the other leg.

2-4. POWER TRAINING

Two kinds of power training are necessary in order to master the sword: muscle power and internal energy.

Muscle Training

Push-Ups. Muscle power is developed by strengthening the fingers, the grip, and the arms. The fingers are strengthened by doing push-ups on the finger tips (Figure 2-13). Work up to twenty repetitions. Endurance is developed by holding the push-up position (Figure 2-14) as long as possible, working up to between one and three minutes.

Bamboo Twisting. The grip is strengthened by working with bundles of bamboo rods with a training partner (Figures 2-15 to 2-17). Both people turn and raise the bundle in opposite directions. Take turns, one person holding the bundle tightly, the other somewhat loosely, and repeat 50 times. This conditions the palms and helps to strengthen the fingers.

Windlass. This exercise is done using a five to ten pound weight suspended with a cord from the center of a short wooden bar. Stand with the feet well apart and hold the bar straight out at shoulder level. Wind the cord onto the bar, thereby lifting the

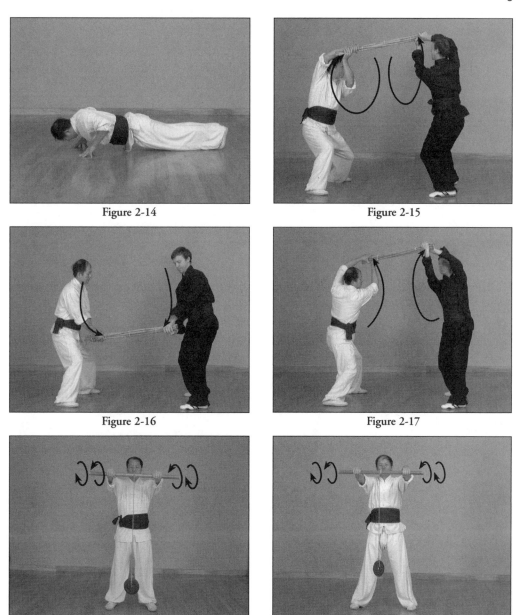

Figure 2-14

Figure 2-15

Figure 2-16

Figure 2-17

Figure 2-18

Figure 2-19

weight as far as it will go. Slowly lower the weight by unwinding the cord, continue winding the cord to lift the weight again, then lower it to the floor. This set should be performed with the hands held palm down as in Figure 2-18, and with the hands held palm up as in Figure 2-19. Practice winding the weight up and down in both directions at least 10 times. Increase the weight as you are able.

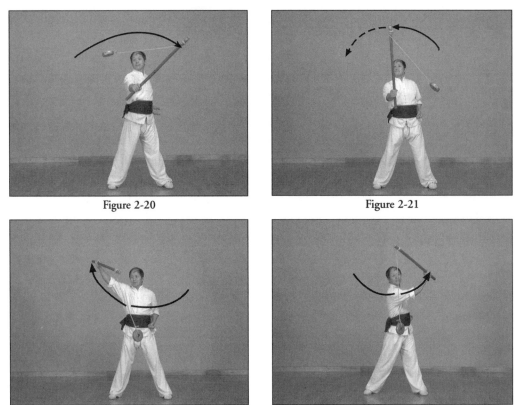

Figure 2-20

Figure 2-21

Figure 2-22

Figure 2-23

Stick Training. These three exercises are done using a thick three foot dowel with a five to ten pound weight suspended from one end. Stand with the feet well apart and hold the stick like a sword. First move the tip from side to side without letting the weight change position and keeping the handle from moving as well (Figures 2-20 and 2-21). This trains the arm for repelling and covering. Next move the handle end from side to side while keeping the weight and tip of the stick stationary (Figures 2-22 and 2-23). This trains the arm for sliding and blocking. Finally, keep the tip of the stick and the weight stationary and move the hand in a three foot circle both clockwise and counterclockwise. This develops strength and suppleness in the arm. Although these are muscle training exercises, if the student concentrates, he can generate internal energy as well.

Accuracy Training. The student can devise his own methods for learning to cut and thrust accurately. An example of a way to practice cutting is to mount two dowels with a narrow space between them as in Figure 2-24. Practice sliding the tip of the sword between the dowels without touching them. The width of the space between them can be varied, and tape can be used to limit the length of the slit as well in order to practice cutting to a particular depth or to practice using the very tip

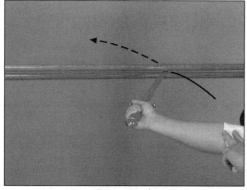

Figure 2-24

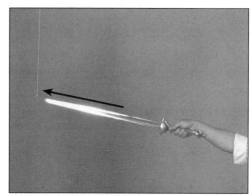

Figure 2-25

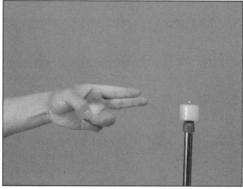

Figure 2-26

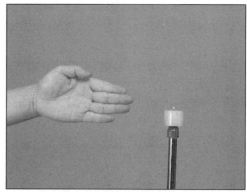

Figure 2-27

of the sword. Stabbing can be practiced by suspending a small object on a long cord and stabbing it, trying to hit it while it swings about (Figure 2-25).

Internal Power Training

In order to use the sword effectively the student must learn to generate internal power (Qi) in his body and project it into the sword, balancing the flow of energy with the secret sword hand. This is extremely difficult. The best way to

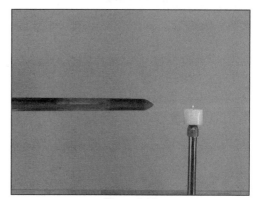

Figure 2-28

develop this energy is to use candle training (Figures 2-26 to 2-28). Hold the hand close to a candle in the finger or palm secret sword. By concentrating, use internal power to bend the flame away. After learning to do this the student then uses the tip of the sword. The student should consult the author's books on Qigong and White Crane martial arts for methods of developing internal power.

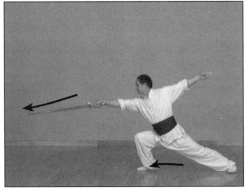

Figure 2-29

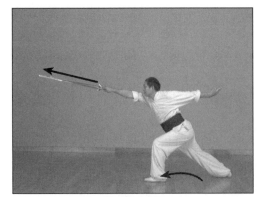

Figure 2-30

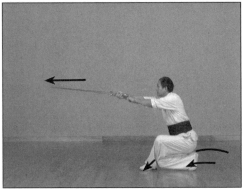

Figure 2-31

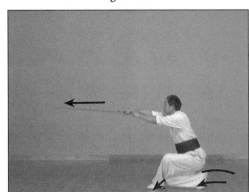

Figure 2-32

2-5. KEY WORDS AND TECHNIQUES

Every style of martial arts has its own unique group of key words and techniques, although most key words and techniques are used by more than one style. A key word describes a technique that is fundamental to the way the style works. The key words and techniques described here are those of the Shaolin Long Fist style.

Stab (Ci, 刺). Stab means to strike with the tip of the sword in a straight thrust. This technique can be performed with the sword blade vertical with the palm facing to the left (Vertical Stab, Zheng Li Ci, 正立刺) (Figure 2-29), with the palm facing right (Reverse Vertical Stab, Fan Li Ci, 反立刺) (Figure 2-30), or with the sword held horizontally either palm up (Horizontal Stab, Zheng Ping Ci, 正平刺) (Figure 2-31) or palm down (Reverse Horizontal Stab, Fan Ping Ci, 反平刺) (Figure 2-32).

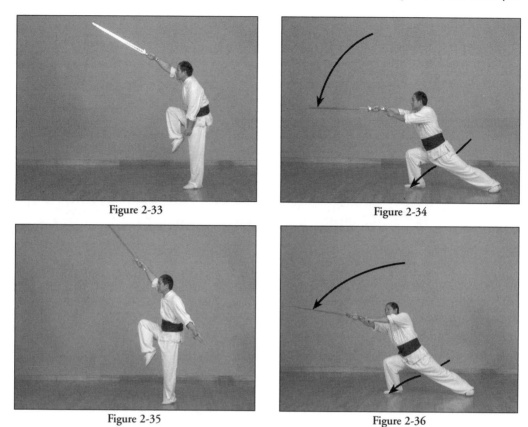

Figure 2-33

Figure 2-34

Figure 2-35

Figure 2-36

Chop or Split (Pi, 劈). Chop or Split means to strike with the edge of the top third of the blade. The motion can be either vertical (Vertical Chop, Zheng Pi, 正劈) (Figures 2-33 and 2-34) or diagonal (Diagonal Chop, Xie Pi, 斜劈) (Figs. 35 and 36).

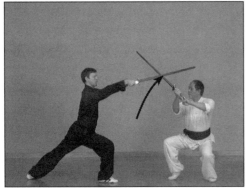

Figure 2-37

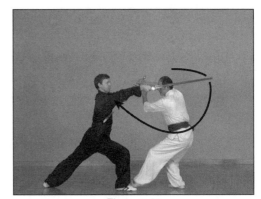

Figure 2-38

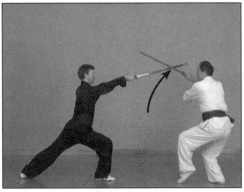

Figure 2-39

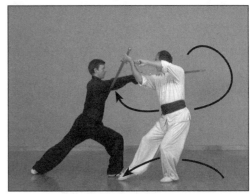

Figure 2-40

Slide Block and Cut (Liao, 撩). Slide Block and Cut means to parry an opponent's chop by sliding it up to the side, then to attack under the opponent's weapon and cut him with the sharp part of the blade by pulling the sword upward. This movement can be performed either to the left (Normal Slide Up, Zheng Liao, 正撩) (Figures 2-37 and 2-38) or the right (Reverse Slide Up, Fan Liao, 反撩) (Figures 2-39 and 2-40).

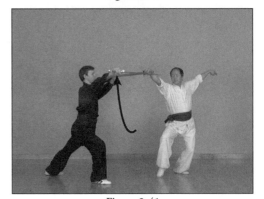

Figure 2-41

Pluck (Tiao, 挑). Pluck (Figure 2-41) means to cut the enemy's wrist by lifting the sword.

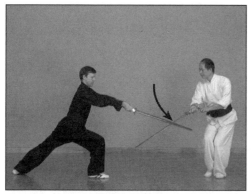

Figure 2-42

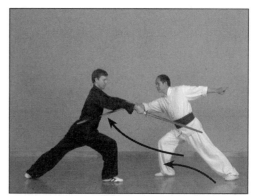

Figure 2-43

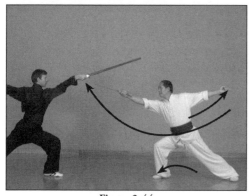

Figure 2-44

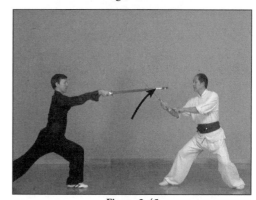

Figure 2-45

Horizontal Extend (Beng, 弸).
Horizontal Extend (Figures 2-42 to 2-44) means to cut the enemy with a backhand horizontal stroke. Against a stab, slide block the enemy's sword to the left, then perform the Horizontal Extend to cut the torso. Against an attack from the rear, turn around to the right and use the Horizontal Extend to cut the enemy's sword wrist (Figure 2-44).

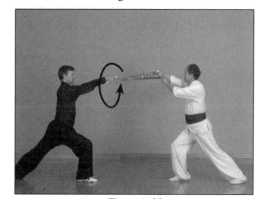

Figure 2-46

Lift (Gua, 掛). Lift means when an enemy stabs or chops at you, you block either to the inside or the outside, and then lift up your sword, slicing the enemy's wrist. If you block to the inside and lift to the enemy's wrist, it is called an External Lift (Wai Shang Gua, 外上掛) (Figures 2-45 and 2-46). If you block to the outside and lift to the enemy's wrist, it is called an Internal Lift (Nei Shang Gua, 內上掛) (Figures 2-47 and 2-48). If you block to the inside, then lift to the enemy's wrist from the outside, it is called an External Reverse Lift (Wai Fan Gua, 外反掛) (Figures 2-49 and 2-50).

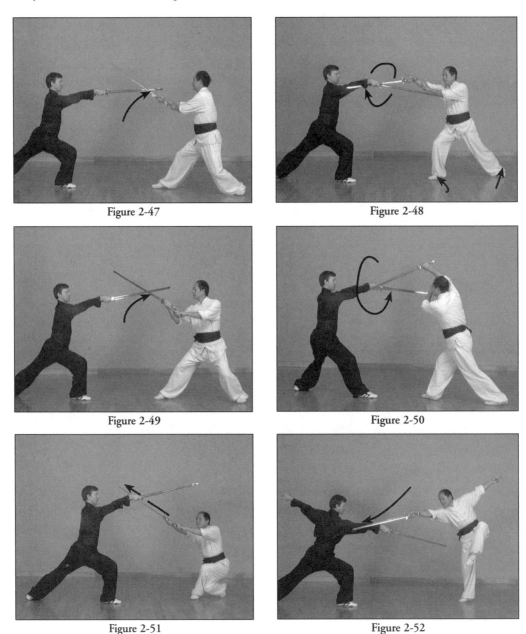

Figure 2-47

Figure 2-48

Figure 2-49

Figure 2-50

Figure 2-51

Figure 2-52

File (Cuo, 挫、錯). File means means to cut by thrusting the sword away from you rather than pulling it toward you. If you file upward, it is called an Upward File (Shang Cuo, 上挫) (Figure 2-51). If you file from the enemy's inside, it is called an Internal File (Nei Cuo, 內挫) (Figure 2-52), and if you file the enemy's wrist from the outside, it is called an External File (Wai Cuo, 外挫) (Figure 2-53).

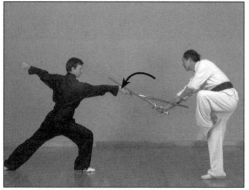

Figure 2-53

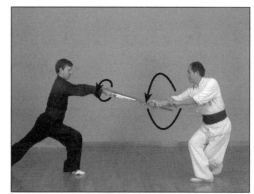

Figure 2-54

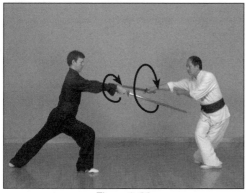

Figure 2-55

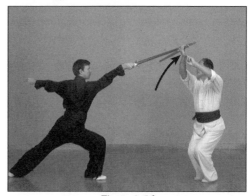

Figure 2-56

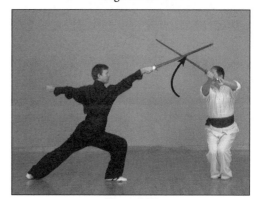

Figure 2-57

Wrap (Jiao, 絞). Wrap is a very frequently used technique in which you evade a cut to your wrist and cut the enemy's wrist by moving the hand in a circle (see Fundamental Training for key techniques below). If you wrap your enemy's wrist from the outside (counterclockwise), it is called an External Wrap (Wai Jiao, 外絞) (Figure 2-54). If you wrap the enemy's wrist from the inside (clockwise), it is called an Internal Wrap (Nei Jiao, 內絞) (Figure 2-55).

Bear (Tuo, 托). Bear is a strong upward or diagonal block with the thick, blunt butt end of the blade. If you block upward, it is called an Upward Bear (Zheng Tuo or Shang Tuo, 正托、上托) (Figure 2-56). If you block diagonally, it is called a Diagonal Bear (Xie Tuo, 斜托) (Figure 2-57).

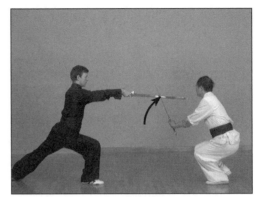

Figure 2-58

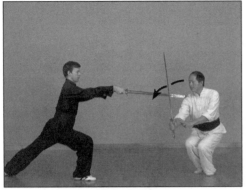

Figure 2-59

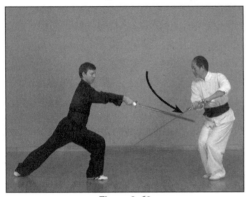

Figure 2-60

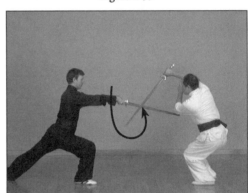

Figure 2-61

Hinder or Obstruct (Lan, 攔). A deflection of a stab by sliding the enemy's weapon to the side away from your body. If you slide block from the inside, it is called an Internal Hinder (Nei Zhong Lan, 內中攔) (Figure 2-58). If you slide block from the outside, it is called an External Hinder (Wai Zhong Lan, 外中攔) (Figure 2-59). If you slide block a low attack internally, it is called a Low Internal Hinder (Nei Xia Lan, 內下攔) (Figure 2-60), and if you block a low attack externally, it is called a Low External Hinder (Wai Xia Lan, 外下攔) (Figure 2-61).

Intercept (Jie, 截). Intercept is a fast chop to the enemy's wrist to intercept a stab. If you chop the enemy's wrist internally, it is called an Internal Intercept (Nei Jie, 內截) (Figure 2-62). If you intercept an attack from the outside, it is called an External Intercept (Wai Jie, 外截) (Figure 2-63). If you intercept an attack from the outside with a low cut, it is called an External Low Intercept (Wai Xia Jie, 外下截) (Figure 2-64), and if you intercept from the inside with a low cut, it is called an Internal Low Intercept (Nei Xia Jie, 內下截) (Figure 2-65).

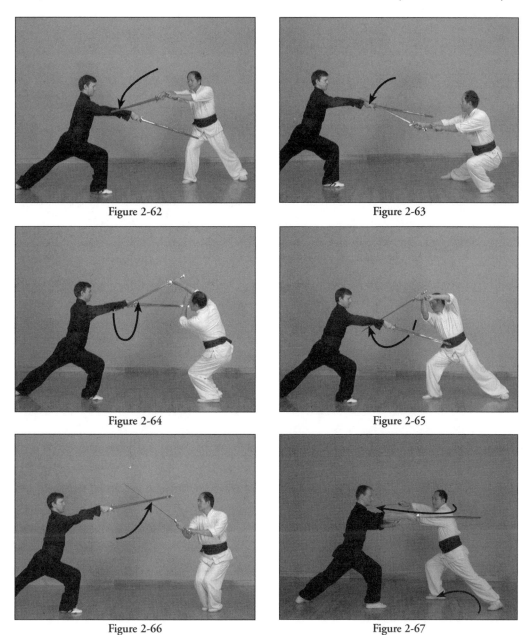

Figure 2-62

Figure 2-63

Figure 2-64

Figure 2-65

Figure 2-66

Figure 2-67

Smear (Mo, 摸**).** Smear is a strong attack to the neck or torso. This is a follow-up to the Hinder technique (above). If you deflect the enemy's attack from the inside and then smear the neck, it is called a High Internal Smear (Shang Nei Mo, 上內摸) (Figures 2-66 and 2-67). If you Hinder the attack from the outside and then smear

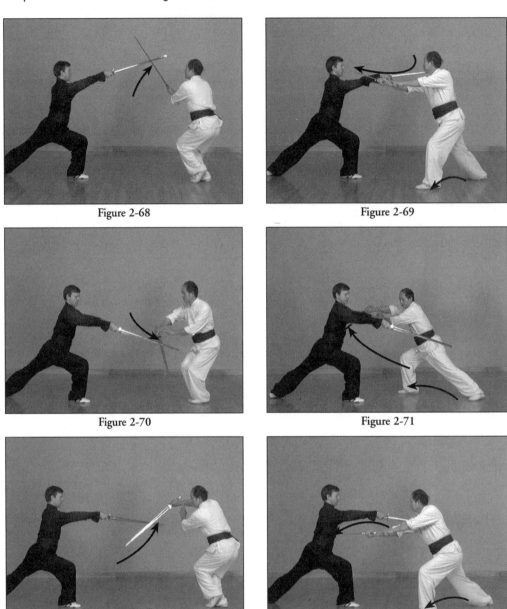

Figure 2-68

Figure 2-69

Figure 2-70

Figure 2-71

Figure 2-72

Figure 2-73

the neck, this is called a High External Smear (Shang Wai Mo, 上外摸) (Figures 2-68 and 2-69). If you deflect the enemy's low attack internally and then smear the stomach, it is called a Low Internal Smear (Xia Nei Mo, 下內摸) (Figures 2-70 and 2-71). However, if you slide block the enemy's low attack externally, it is called a Low External Smear (Xia Wai Mo, 下外摸) (Figures 2-72 and 2-73).

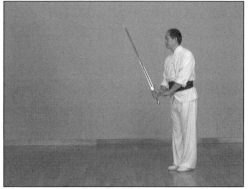

Figure 2-74

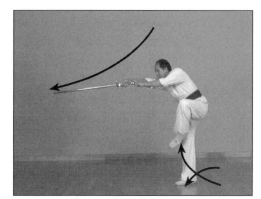

Figure 2-75

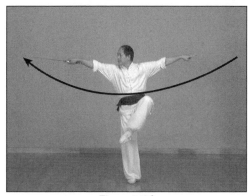

Figure 2-76

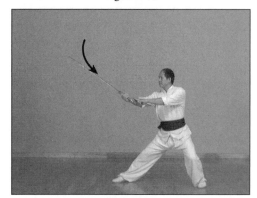

Figure 2-77

Point (Dian, 點). Point (Figures 2-74 and 2-75) is a stabbing technique in which the point of the sword is directed downward as it enters the enemy's body. This makes it easier to withdraw the sword.

Cloud (Yun, 雲). Cloud (Figure 2-76) is mainly a defensive move to keep an opponent at a distance. It is a back-handed high cut executed by turning around with the sword extended.

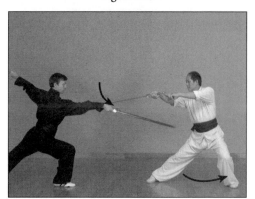

Figure 2-78

Draw Back (Le, 将). Draw Back means to slide the sword across the enemy's wrist while withdrawing. If you draw back from inside, it is called an Internal Draw Back (Nei Le, 內将) (Figures 2-77 and 2-78). If you draw back outside, it is called an External Draw Back (Wai Le, 外将) (Figures 2-79 and 2-80).

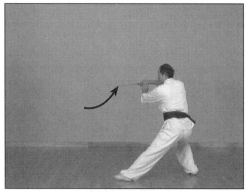

Figure 2-79

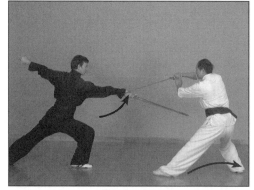

Figure 2-80

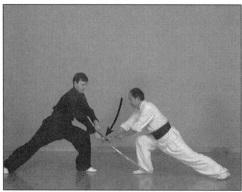

Figure 2-81

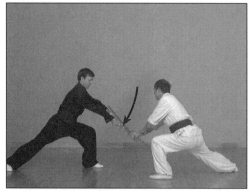

Figure 2-82

Cover (**Gai**, 蓋). Cover means to block the opponent's weapon and immobilize it with a forward and downward push. If you cover from the inside, it is called an Internal Cover (Nei Gai, 內蓋) (Figure 2-81). If you cover from the outside, it is called an External Cover (Wai Gai, 外蓋) (Figure 2-82).

Block Upward (**Ge**, 格). Block Upward(Figure 2-83) is a strong block like Bear (above), except that the sword is held backhanded, with the palm facing upward.

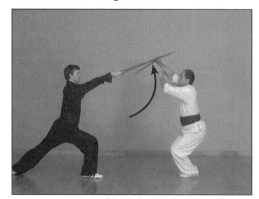

Figure 2-83

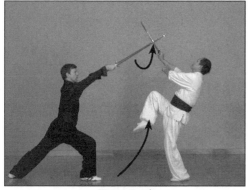

Figure 2-84

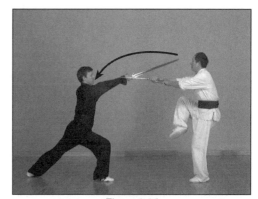

Figure 2-85

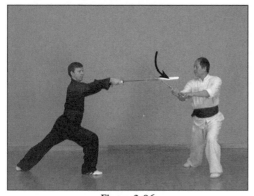

Figure 2-86

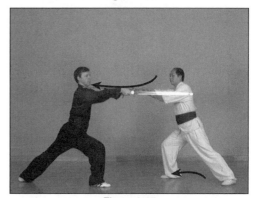

Figure 2-87

Wash (Xi, 洗). Wash (Figures 2-84 and 2-85) means to deflect the opponent's sword to the side then cut to the neck with one circular motion.

Shake (Yao, 搖). Shake (Figures 2-86 and 2-87) means to hold the sword blade horizontal with the palm facing up and shake the blade from side to side to block or to cut the opponent while moving either forward or backward.

Rise (Jie, 揭). Rise (Figure 2-88)

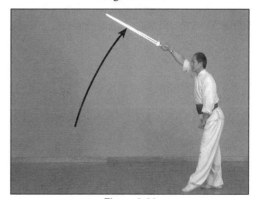

Figure 2-88

means to block the opponent's weapon straight up, then attack by chopping straight down.

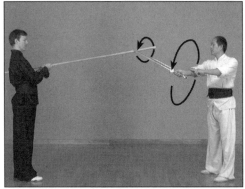

Figure 2-89

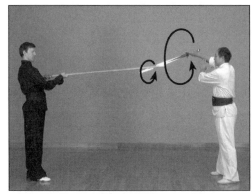

Figure 2-90

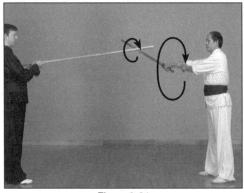

Figure 2-91

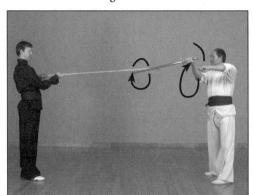

Figure 2-92

2-6. FUNDAMENTAL TRAINING

In order to understand and master the key word techniques presented above the student must practice them. The basic practice routines are given below.

Wrap Hand. Keep the sword point in one spot and rotate the sword hand in one-foot circles, both counterclockwise (Figures 2-89 and 2-90) and clockwise (Figures 2-91 and 2-92).

Slide Block and Cut. Deflect to the side in the taming the tiger stance, then step forward into the crossed leg stance and cut to the knee (Figures 2-93 and 2-94). Continue the movement either forward or backward.

Hinder or Obstruct. Deflect to one side in the golden rooster stance, then hop to the other foot into the golden rooster stance and deflect to the other side (Figures 2-95 and 2-96).

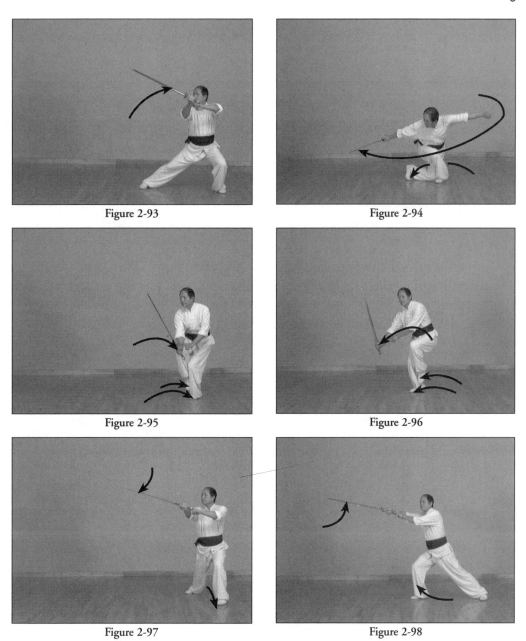

Figure 2-93

Figure 2-94

Figure 2-95

Figure 2-96

Figure 2-97

Figure 2-98

Shake. Walk forward and backward while moving the sword from side to side in coordination with the footwork (Figures 2-97 and 2-98). The sword should move in the same direction as the forward foot when walking forward and the reverse when walking backward.

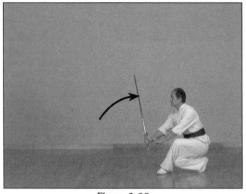

Figure 2-99

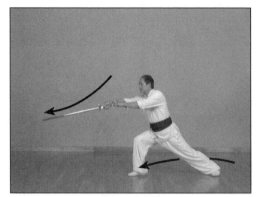

Figure 2-100

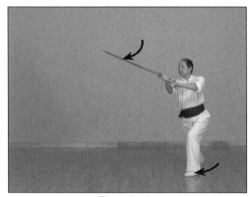

Figure 2-101

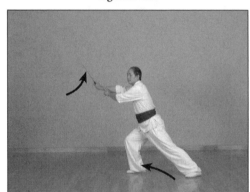

Figure 2-102

Walking Point. Walk forward or backward. With each step stab forward and downward, then bring the sword to a ready position (Figure 2-99) and step and point again (Figures 2-100).

Hinder or Obstruct. Step forward and to the side while deflecting to the same side (Figures 2-101 and 2-102). Practice side to side, forward and backward.

Slide up. Stand still and move the sword in a figure eight, first blocking upward to one side, then sliding up to the other (Figures 2-103 to 2-106).

Jumping Point. Lunge forward, stabbing slightly downward. Withdraw the sword by flicking the point upward (Figures 2-107 and 2-108). Repeat the movement, moving either forward or backward.

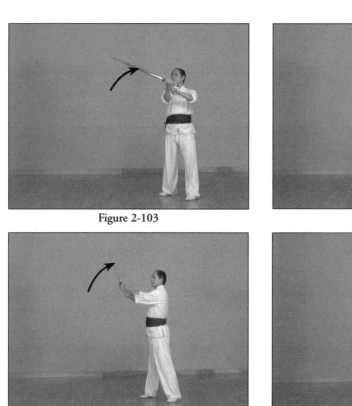

Figure 2-103

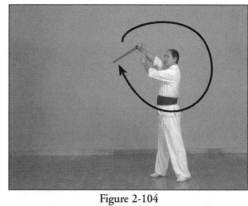

Figure 2-104

Figure 2-105

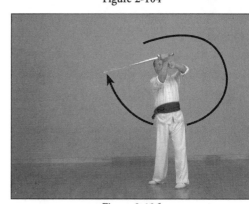

Figure 2-106

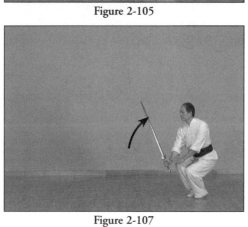

Figure 2-107

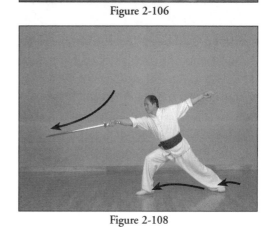

Figure 2-108

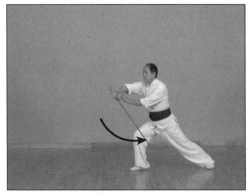

Figure 2-109

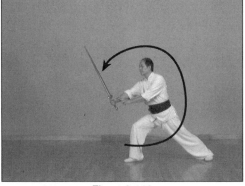

Figure 2-110

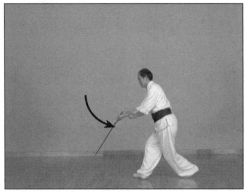

Figure 2-111

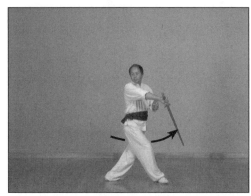

Figure 2-112

Slide Cut Left, Block Right, Turn Around and Chop. Slide cut to the left while standing in bow and arrow stance (Figures 2-109 and 2-110), then turn to the right into a high crossed leg stance blocking (Figure 2-111); finally turn to the right again hopping into a golden rooster stance while chopping forward (Figures 2-112 and 2-113). Repeat the sequence.

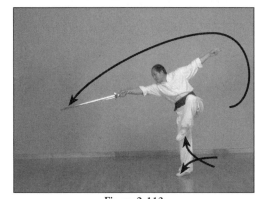

Figure 2-113

CHAPTER 3

San Cai Jian
三才劍

3-1. INTRODUCTION

"San Cai Jian" (三才劍) means "The Three Powers Sword Sequence." "San Cai" refers in Chinese culture to the three powers of heaven (Tian, 天), earth (Di, 地), and man (Ren, 人).

No one knows when or by whom the San Cai Jian sequence was created. It is said that this sequence was first passed down during the Qing Dynasty (1644-1911 A.D., 清朝) by Li, Cai-Ting (李彩亭) who lived at Ding Xing Xian in Hebei Province (河北、定興縣). This sequence introduces the basic techniques and principles of sword. It not only helps the beginner to build a foundation of sword skills and to understand the principles of sword technique, but it also introduces the beginner to applying Qi to weapons. This sequence has been famous in China and was a required sequence in the two largest martial institutions there; the Nanking Central Guoshu Institute (南京中央國術館) (founded in 1928), and the Jing Wu Association (上海精武體育會) (founded in 1909). However, many Chinese martial artists believe that this sequence originated in Xingyiquan style, and has been passed down since ancient times.

The most important and unique characteristic of this sequence is that the techniques of the first part of the sequence match those of the second part. It is the only known sword sequence that matches itself, so that it can be practiced by two people. Like a musical round, one person starts the first part, while the second person starts the second. The primary counterattacks in this sequence focus on the wrist, so that it is possible for two people to practice it with sharp swords without risk of serious injury. However, the reader should understand that it is much harder to attack the wrist than the body. If a person can skillfully attack an enemy's wrist, he should have no problem inflicting a more serious injury on the opponent's body.

3-2. SAN CAI JIAN 三才劍

This sequence will be introduced with the pictures of the matching forms and the corresponding solo forms for both performers. The number of the solo form pictures will match those of the matching form pictures, and will be identified as 1W, 2W,...etc. for the performer with the white shirt, and 1B, 2B,...etc. for the performer with the black shirt.

When solo forms are practiced, the student should first do from 1W to 95W (white performer) for the first part and continue from 15B to the end (black performer) for the second part. In the same way, when matching forms are performed, one practitioner should first do the 1W to 95W and then continue from 15B to the end. His partner should start with 1B to 95B, and then 20W to the end. The student should end the sequence on the same spot he started from. Most Chinese martial sequences are designed this way. When a student begins a sequence, he faces the master or the audience; when he finishes, out of politeness and respect, he should end with the same orientation and position.

In this chapter, the matching forms will explain the first level application only. No second level or deeper solution will be given. In the captions "White" represents the person wearing the white shirt, while "Black" represents the person wearing the black shirt.

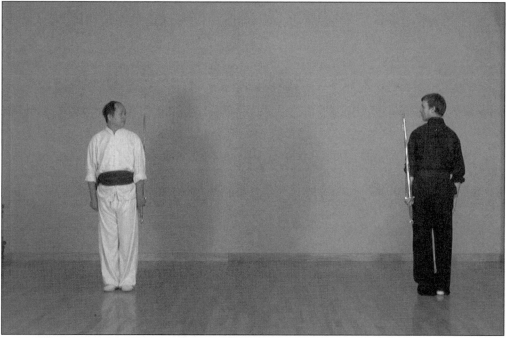

Figure 3-1

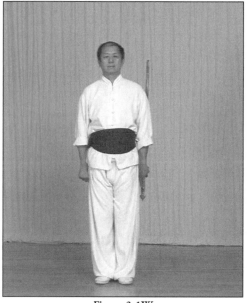

Figure 3-1W

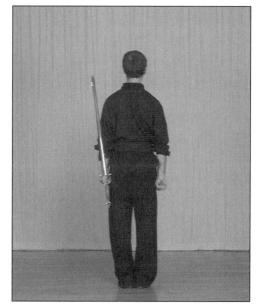

Figure 3-1B

Figure 3-1: White begins with the body facing north while Black stands the same way with the body facing south. The sword is held in the left hand, palms to the rear as shown. For solo practice, the head looks forward.

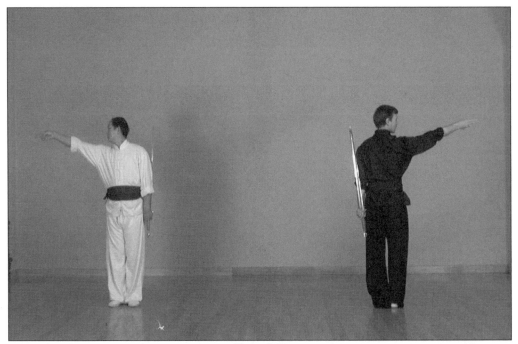

Figure 3-2

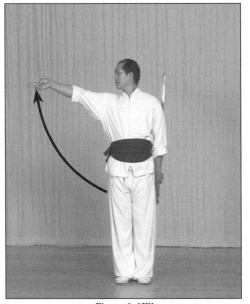

Figure 3-2W

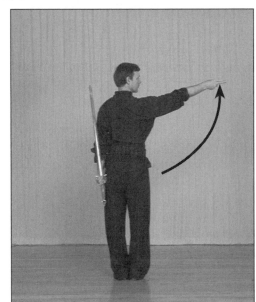

Figure 3-2B

Figure 3-2: Both White and Black look to their right as they raise their right arms up from the side and point the first and second fingers to the right, palm forward.

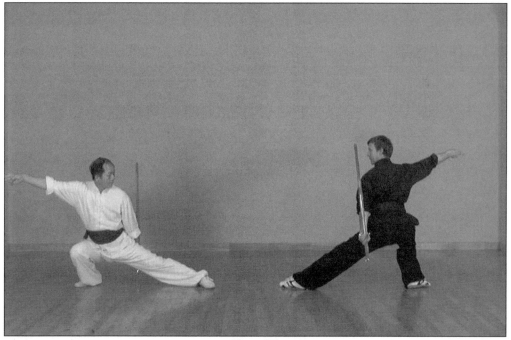

Figure 3-3

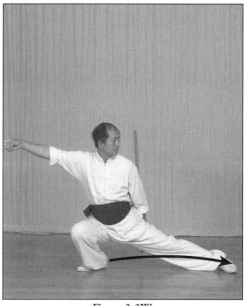

Figure 3-3W

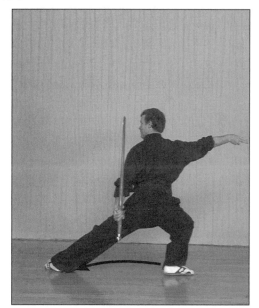

Figure 3-3B

Figure 3-3: Both White and Black step to their left in the taming the tiger stance, looking at each other.

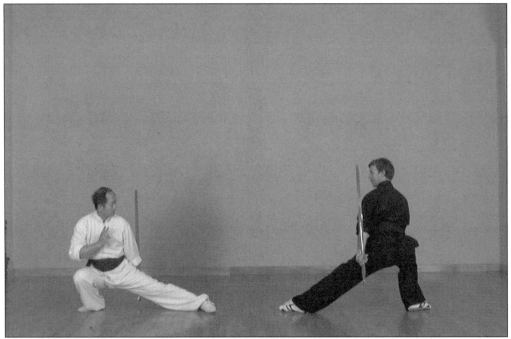

Figure 3-4

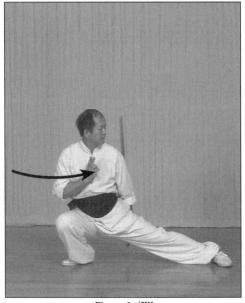

Figure 3-4W

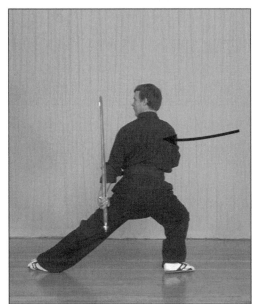

Figure 3-4B

Figure 3-4: Keeping the same stance, both White and Black bring their right hands to their chests with the first and second fingers pointing upward.

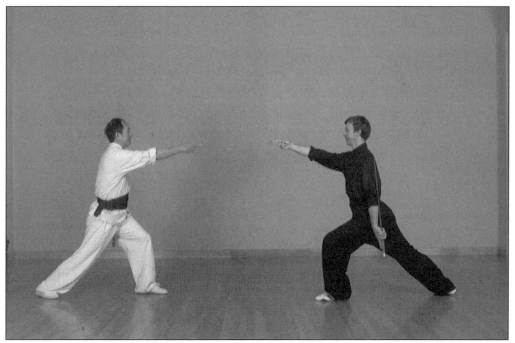

Figure 3-5

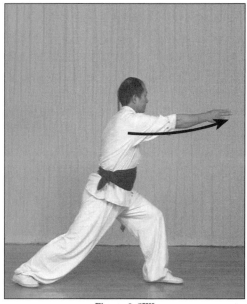

Figure 3-5W

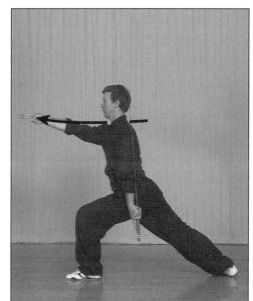

Figure 3-5B

Figure 3-5: Both White and Black change their stance to the bow and arrow stance with the left foot forward. As they change their stances, their right hands move forward from the chest and point toward each other. Their left arms have not moved thus far.

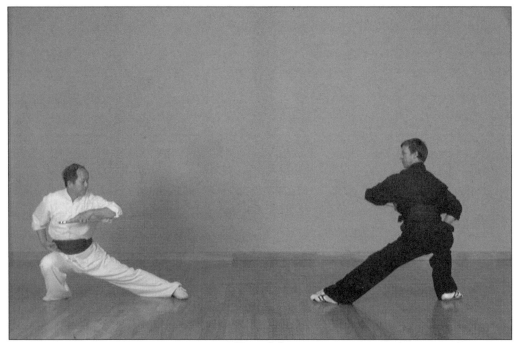

Figure 3-6

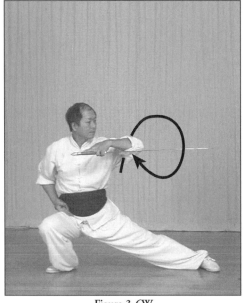

Figure 3-6W

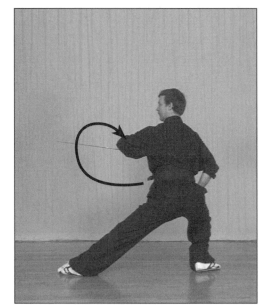

Figure 3-6B

Figure 3-6: Both White and Black sit back again in the taming the tiger stance as shown. As they move back, the left arm, which is holding the sword, moves across the chest with the palm down. The right hand returns to the waist. White and Black still look at each other.

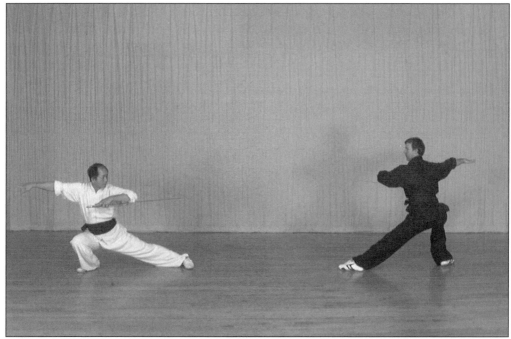

Figure 3-7

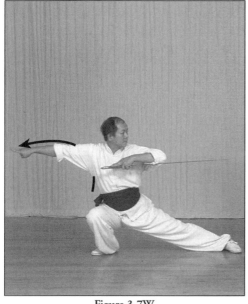

Figure 3-7W

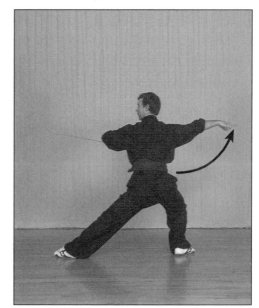

Figure 3-7B

Figure 3-7: White and Black both raise their right hands from the waist in a smooth upward motion to the position shown.

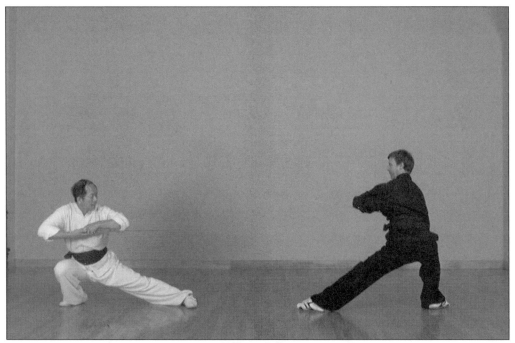

Figure 3-8

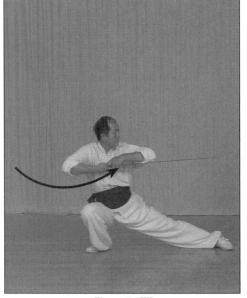

Figure 3-8W

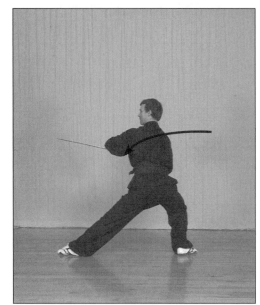

Figure 3-8B

Figure 3-8: Continuing the motion, the right hand moves directly to the other hand and grasps the sword handle.

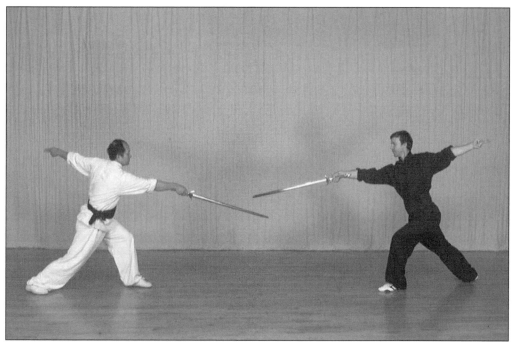

Figure 3-9

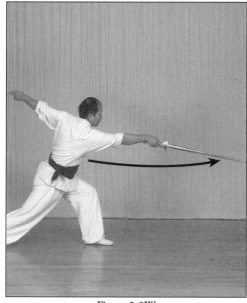

Figure 3-9W

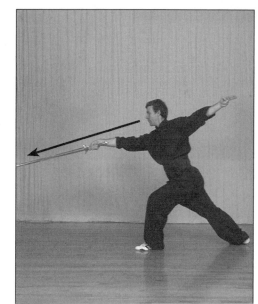

Figure 3-9B

Figure 3-9: Both White and Black move into the bow and arrow stance with the left leg forward. At the same time, each thrusts his sword forward toward the other's midsection. The left hand stretches to the rear as the swords thrust forward.

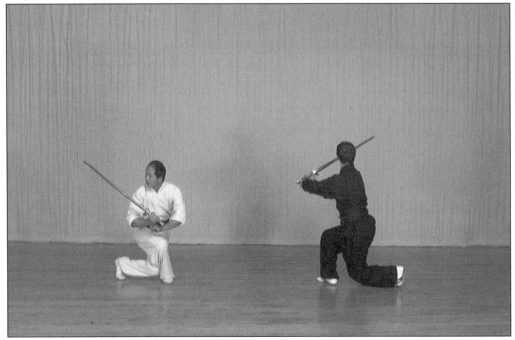

Figure 3-10

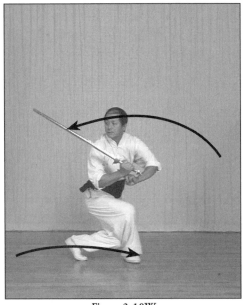

Figure 3-10W

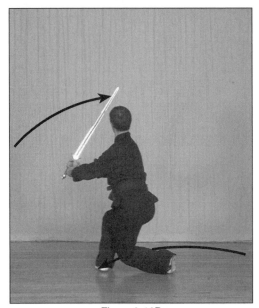

Figure 3-10B

Figure 3-10: Both White and Black then step forward with the right leg into the crossed leg stance as their swords are brought back to the chest and to the right as shown. As this happens, the left hand's two fingers move to the right wrist. Both White and Black look behind them.

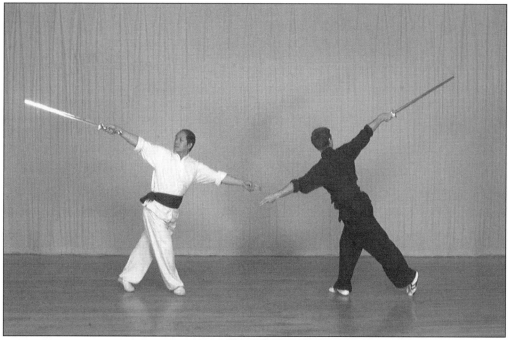

Figure 3-11

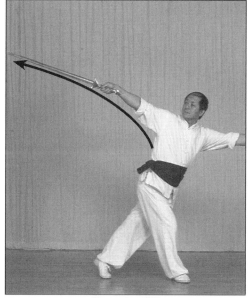

Figure 3-11W

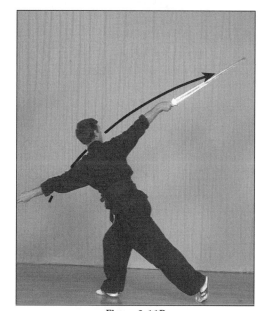

Figure 3-11B

Figure 3-11: Both White and Black change their stances by standing and applying most of the weight to the front (right) leg. The left foot touches with the toes only. As the stance changes, both White and Black thrust their swords to the rear and up while the left hands move forward and down.

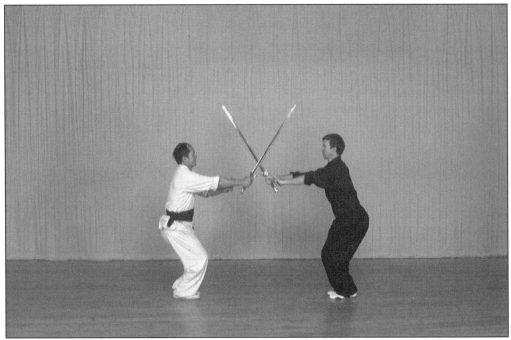

Figure 3-12

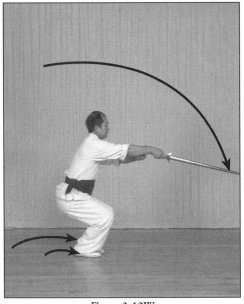

Figure 3-12W

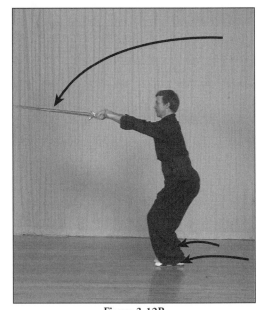

Figure 3-12B

Figure 3-12: Both White and Black then step forward with the left leg, and then move their right feet up next to the left in a second motion. As these steps occur, the sword moves from the rear in a vertical plane over the right shoulder into the position shown, where the right wrist joins the two fingers of the left hand.

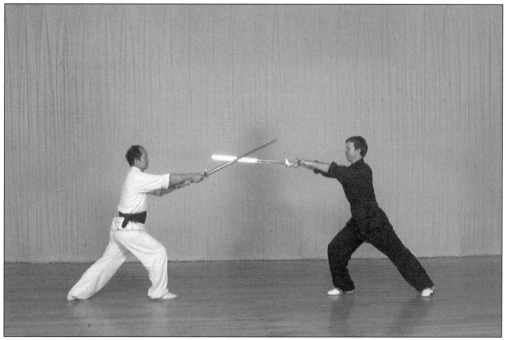

Figure 3-13

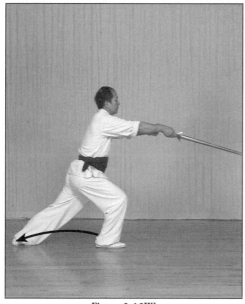

Figure 3-13W

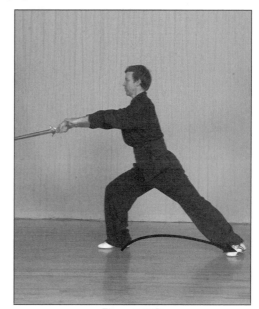

Figure 3-13B

Figure 3-13: Both White and Black step back with the left leg into the bow and arrow stance.

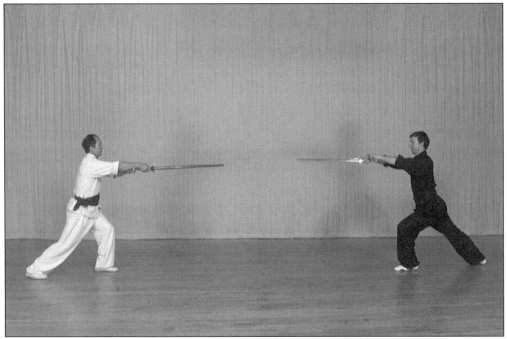

Figure 3-14

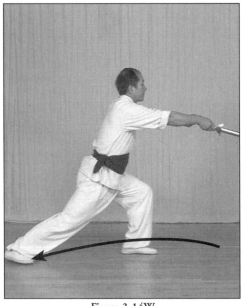

Figure 3-14W

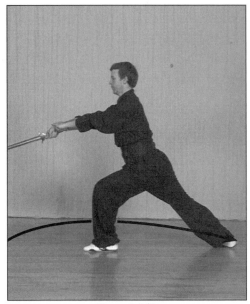

Figure 3-14B

Figure 3-14: Continuing this motion, both White and Black take another step back with the right leg, again ending in the bow and arrow stance.

Figure 3-15: Both White and Black then for the third step bring the left leg back beside the right and stand upright. As this last step occurs, the right hand and sword

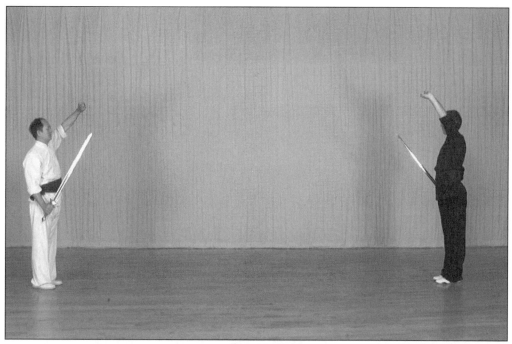

Figure 3-15

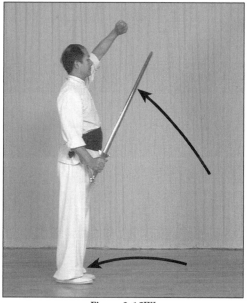
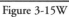

Figure 3-15W

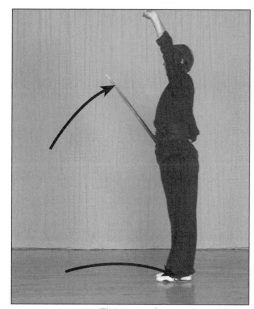

Figure 3-15B

withdraw back to the waist, and the left hand moves up and over the head. The left hand's first and second fingers point to the right. White is facing west and Black is facing east.

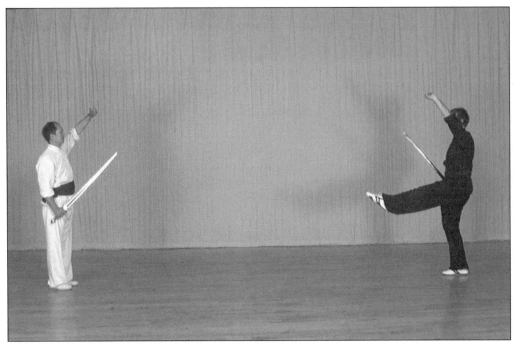

Figure 3-16

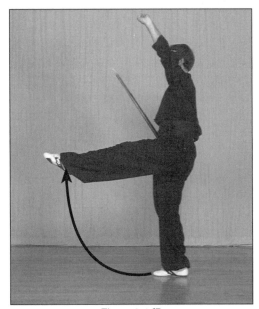

Figure 3-16B

Figures 3-16 and 3-17: Black raises his left foot straight out, up, and back in, as he prepares to attack White.

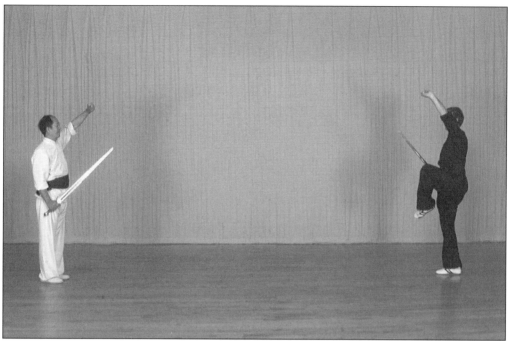

Figure 3-17

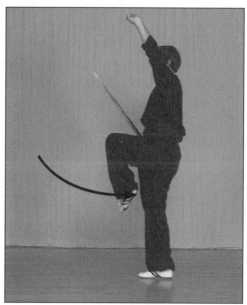

Figure 3-17B

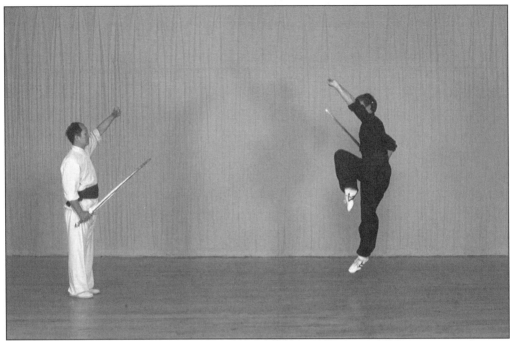

Figure 3-18

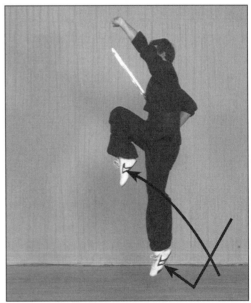

Figure 3-18B

Figure 3-18: Black steps down and forward with his left foot and jumps up, bringing the right knee up, and moves east toward White in the air.

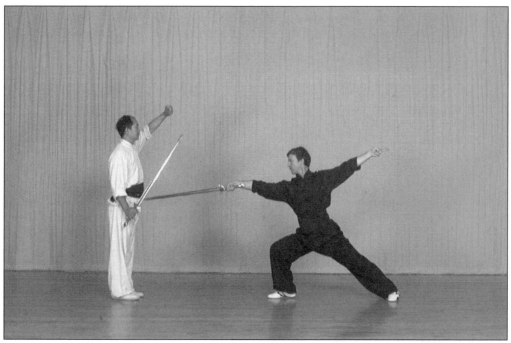

Figure 3-19

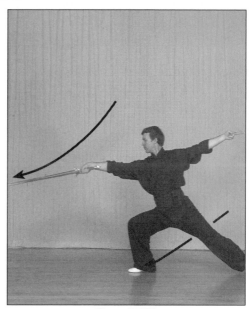

Figure 3-19B

Figure 3-19: Black lands with the right leg forward in the bow and arrow stance and attacks White's midsection. Black's secret sword points west.

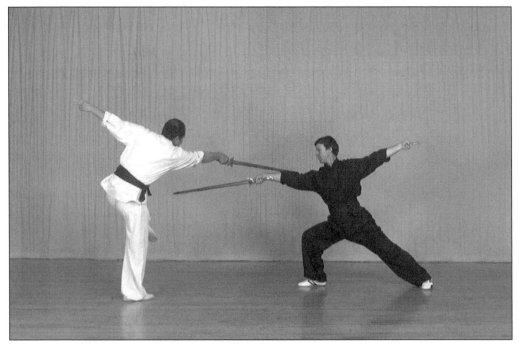

Figure 3-20

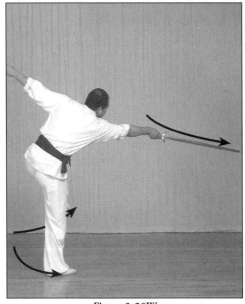

Figure 3-20W

Figure 3-20: As Black attacks White in 19, White avoids the attack by stepping to the northwest as Black's sword comes toward him. White raises his left leg as shown, while he leans his body forward and slices the top of Black's wrist. White's left hand points in the opposite direction from his sword, with the first and second fingers extended.

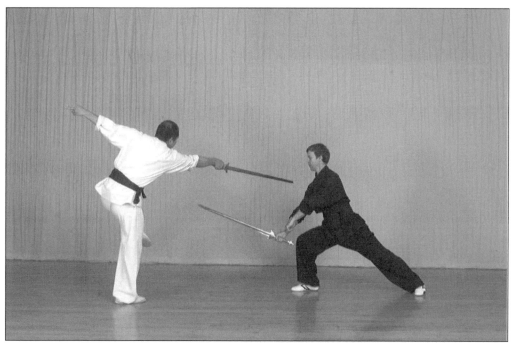

Figure 3-21

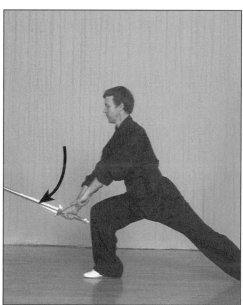

Figure 3-21B

Figure 3-21: As White attacks in Figure 3-20, Black merely drops his wrist down and moves his left hand's two fingers to his right wrist.

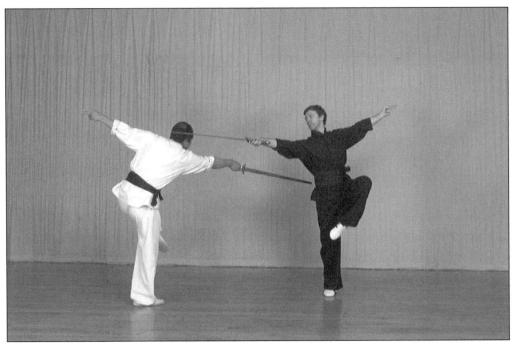

Figure 3-22

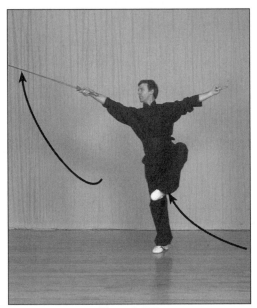

Figure 3-22B

Figure 3-22: Continuing the previous form, Black moves the sword out to the left and back in to cut White's head. At the same time Black raises his left leg. Black's left hand simultaneously extends to his left (west).

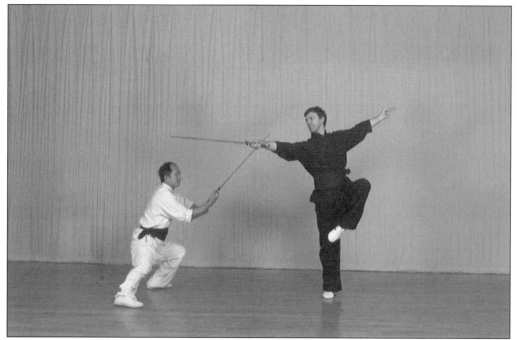

Figure 3-23

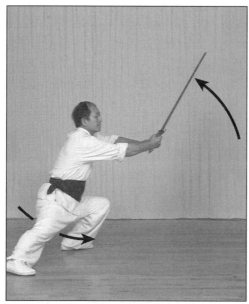

Figure 3-23W

Figure 3-23: White avoids Black's attack to the head by stepping low and to the left (south) into the taming the tiger stance. At the same time, White merely moves his sword from its previous position directly toward Black's wrist. Note also that White's left hand returns to his right wrist with the right palm upward.

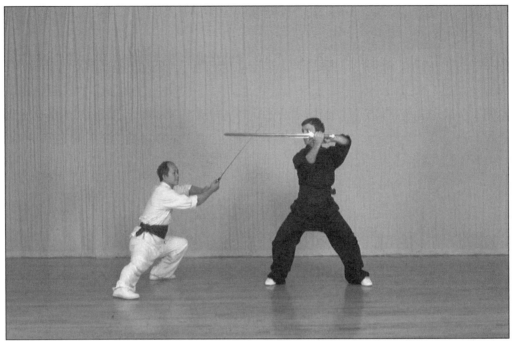

Figure 3-24

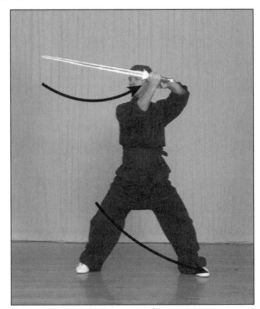

Figure 3-24B

Figure 3-24: To avoid his wrist's being cut, Black steps down into the horse stance and withdraws his sword to a position in front of his chest. Black's left hand moves to the right wrist as this occurs.

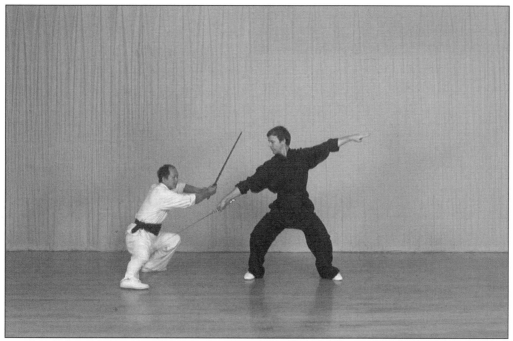

Figure 3-25

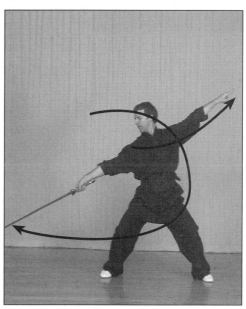

Figure 3-25B

Figure 3-25: After avoiding White's attack, Black remains in the horse stance and cuts down at White's outstretched leg by moving the sword in a counterclockwise circle. Black's left hand moves to his left (west). Both palms face downward.

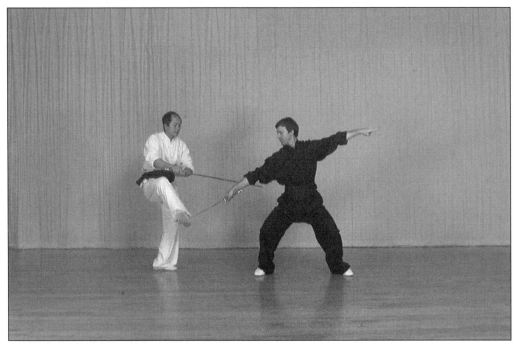

Figure 3-26

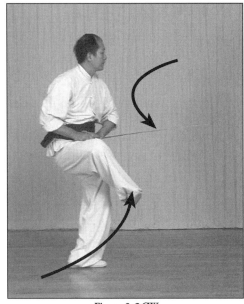

Figure 3-26W

Figure 3-26: To avoid getting his leg cut, White raises his right foot and uses his heel to stop Black's attack as Black's sword approaches. As White blocks with his foot, he turns his right wrist counterclockwise until his palm faces down; at the same time the sword makes a natural counterclockwise circle until White cuts Black's wrist. As

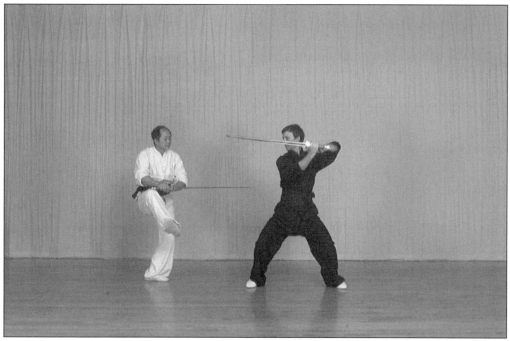

Figure 3-27

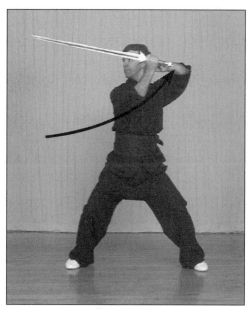

Figure 3-27B

the sword turns to cut Black, White also withdraws his arms in toward his body. White ends facing west, and Black north.

Figure 3-27: Black avoids getting his wrist cut in Figure 3-26 by withdrawing his sword to the chest, rotating his wrist clockwise. The left hand moves to the right wrist.

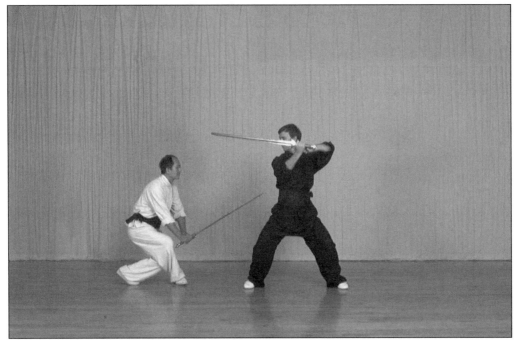

Figure 3-28

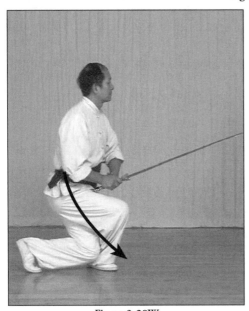

Figure 3-28W

Figure 3-28: White follows Black's retreating motion by moving his right foot forward, facing west, into unicorn stance and thrusting the sword forward, palm downward.

Figure 3-29: Black avoids White's thrust by turning 180 degrees clockwise to face south, moving the right leg into the taming the tiger stance, left leg toward White.

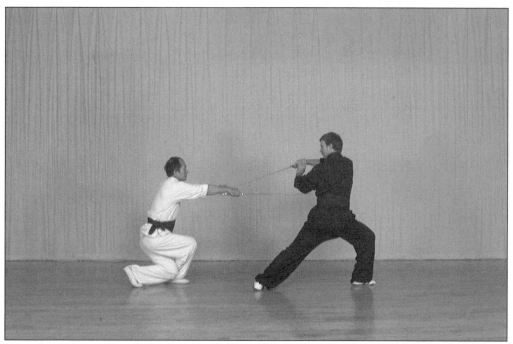

Figure 3-29

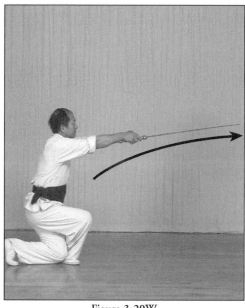

Figure 3-29W

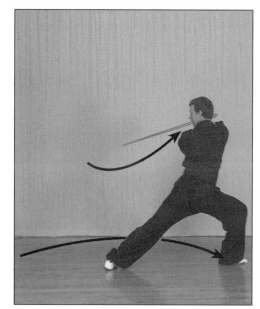

Figure 3-29B

As Black steps back and turns his body clockwise, he twists his sword counterclockwise, tip down, to cut White's wrist as his arms thrust forward. Black's palms are down. To avoid White's attack, Black's arms are above White's sword. White faces west, Black faces south.

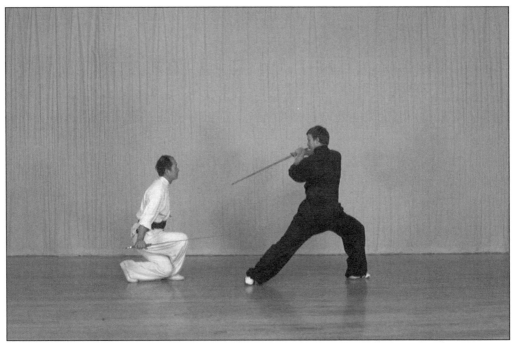

Figure 3-30

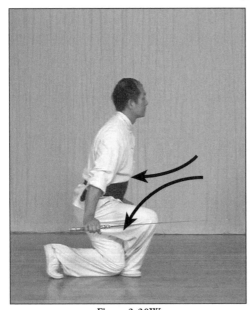

Figure 3-30W

Figure 3-30: White avoids the above attack to his wrist by simply dropping his arms to the sides, palms down, as shown.

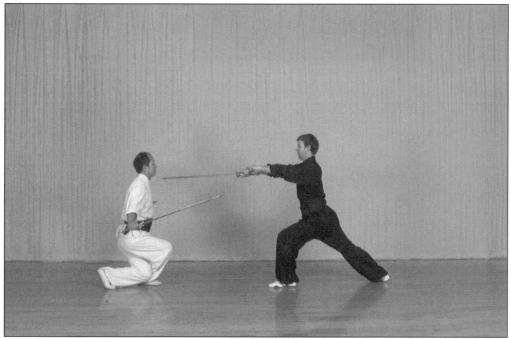

Figure 3-31

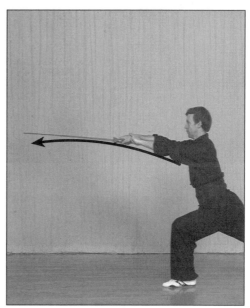

Figure 3-31B

Figure 3-31: Black, noticing White's open position, thrusts forward with his sword, palms down, as he changes his stance to the bow and arrow stance. The left leg is forward, and both arms are extended forward.

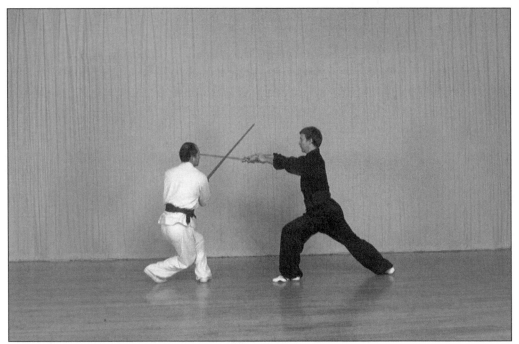

Figure 3-32

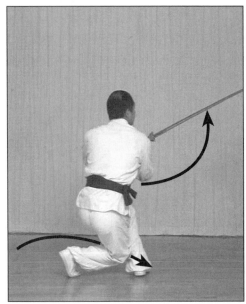

Figure 3-32W

Figure 3-32: Seeing Black's attack coming, White steps forward (west) into the crossed leg stance with his left leg forward. As White steps, he brings the sword up and to the left across his chest as he twists his wrist and sword clockwise. As he steps down into the crossed leg stance, White's left hand returns to the right wrist and his

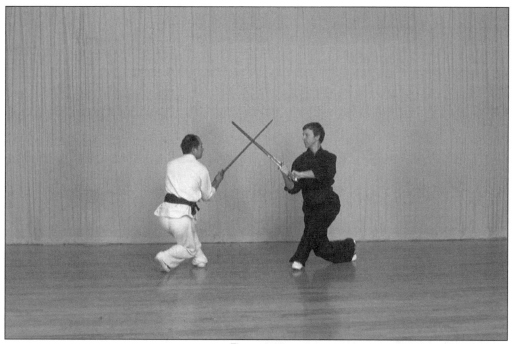

Figure 3-33

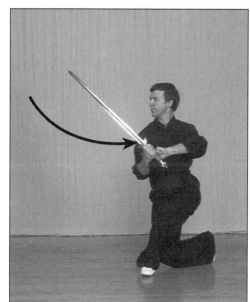

Figure 3-33B

body twists to the left as his sword blocks Black's attack and guides the attack to the side.

Figure 3-33: Black, seeing his vulnerable position, also twists his body to the left and sits down into the crossed leg stance. As he turns, Black turns his wrist clockwise and brings his right elbow back to his chest. By doing this, Black guides White's sword to the left side (north) and protects himself from a potential attack.

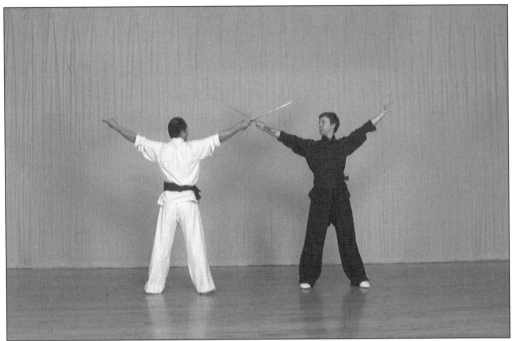

Figure 3-34

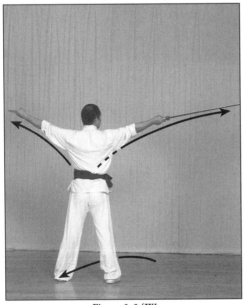

Figure 3-34W

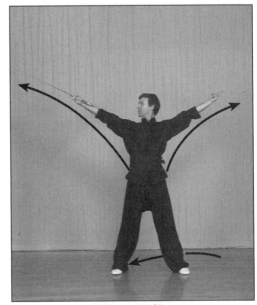

Figure 3-34B

Figure 3-34: Both Black and White, being in the same position, thrust toward each others' heads at the same time as White steps backward with the left foot and Black steps forward with the right foot (White faces south, Black faces north). The result is a double block as shown with the left arms pointing in the opposite directions. Both Black and White stand upright with palms held upward.

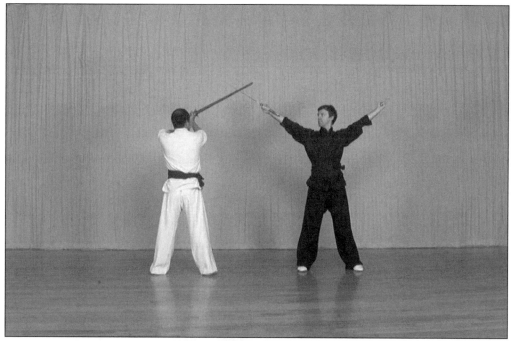

Figure 3-35

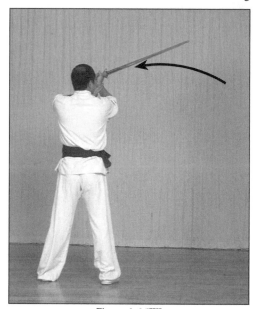

Figure 3-35W

Figure 3-35: White makes the first move by bringing his two hands together at the chest and twisting his right hand clockwise to face himself. White's sword at the same time stays in contact with Black's sword by sliding toward the tip of Black's sword (White's chest faces south).

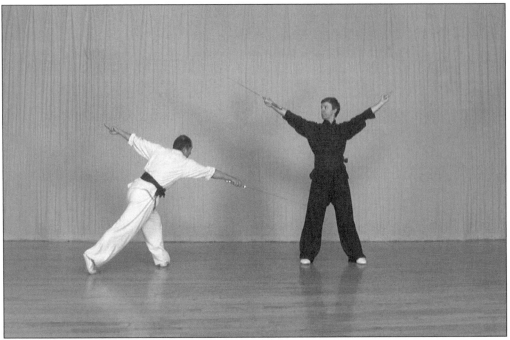

Figure 3-36

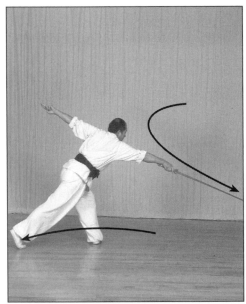

Figure 3-36W

Figure 3-36: Continuing in the same motion, White slides his sword off Black's sword and steps back with his right foot to the northeast touching with the toes only as shown, with most of the weight resting on the left leg. As White steps back, he twists his right wrist counterclockwise so the sword moves smoothly to the left,

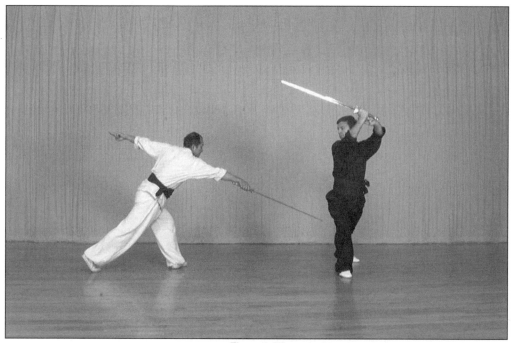

Figure 3-37

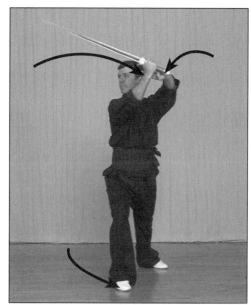

Figure 3-37B

down, and then at a 45 degree angle to cut Black's right leg. As White strikes, his left hand points in the opposite direction from the sword. Note: White steps away from Black because of his vulnerable position in Figure 3-35. To attack without being himself cut first, White would either have to move in and slice Black with his sword or step back and cut as is done here.

Figure 3-37: To avoid White's attack on his right leg, Black steps forward (north) with his right leg away from White's sword, and brings his hands together over his head with the sword pointing toward White. Black's weight is moving toward the right leg, with only the left toes touching the ground.

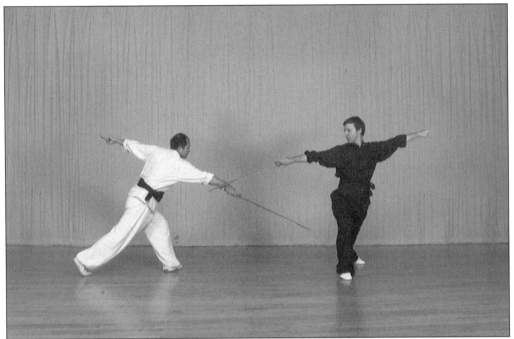

Figure 3-38

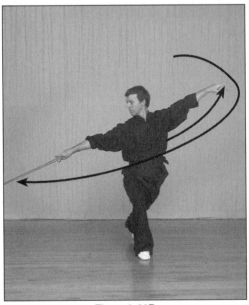

Figure 3-38B

Figure 3-38: Continuing the same motion, Black sets most of his weight down on the right leg with the left toes touching the ground. At the same time Black twists his right hand counterclockwise as the sword travels in a smooth circle up, to the left, and then slashing to the right to cut White's wrist. Black's left hand points in the opposite direction from his sword. Black faces north.

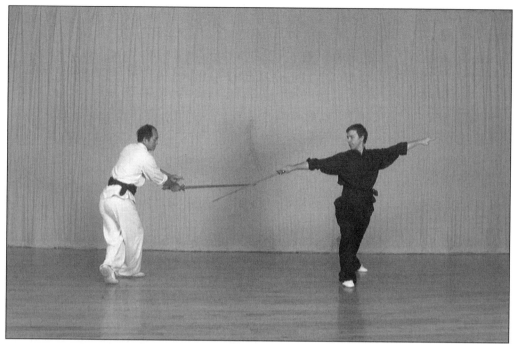

Figure 3-39

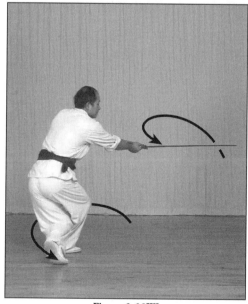

Figure 3-39W

Figure 3-39: To avoid Black's attack on his wrist, White twists his hand clockwise and withdraws his sword toward his chest, palm held upward. As he withdraws his sword, White steps back (north) with the left foot as shown. The left foot actually goes behind and to the right of the right foot, resulting in a crossed leg stance.

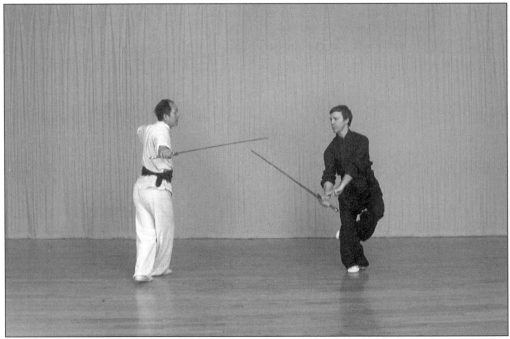

Figure 3-40

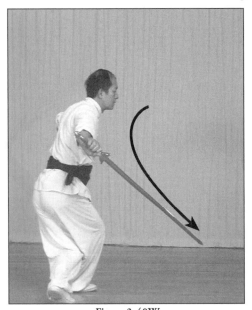

Figure 3-40W

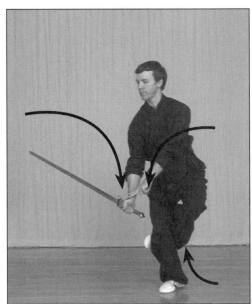

Figure 3-40B

Figure 3-40: White continues the above motion by spreading his arms apart, down, and out as shown, with the right wrist turning counterclockwise, palm down and outward. As White makes his sidestepping advance toward him, Black shifts all his weight to his right leg and puts his left foot behind his right knee. As he does this,

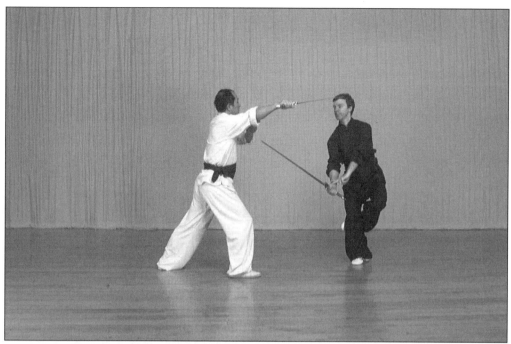

Figure 3-41

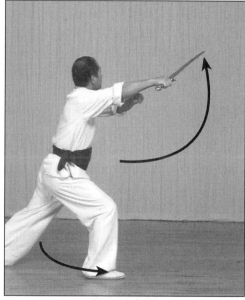

Figure 3-41W

Black turns his right wrist clockwise and brings both hands in front of the body ending up with his right palm facing left; the sword points downward to the north.

Figure 3-41: Again continuing the same motion, White's sword continues its counterclockwise motion by swinging up and wide to the right, keeping the right arm straight and the sword horizontal. The left fingers return to the right wrist. At the same time White steps to the west with his right foot into the bow and arrow stance, facing west. White is now positioned to the northeast of Black. With his right arm straight White thrusts his sword, palm down, toward Black's head with a horizontal counterclockwise motion.

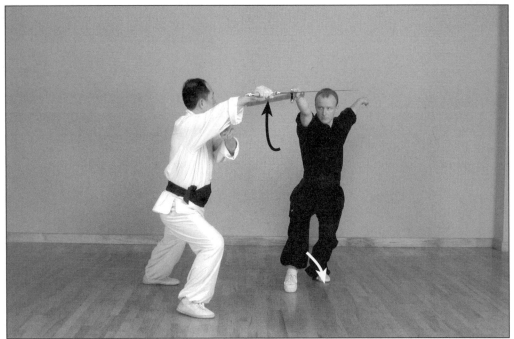

Figure 3-42

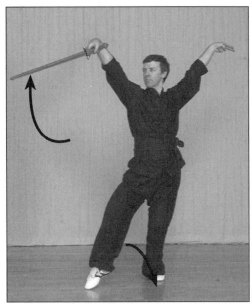

Figure 3-42B

Figure 3-42: Black avoids White's attack to his head by ducking back into the false stance and raising his sword straight up to cut the underside of White's wrist. Black's left hand moves in the opposite direction. Black ends facing north.

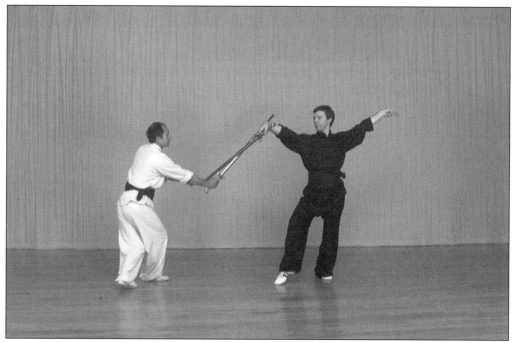

Figure 3-43

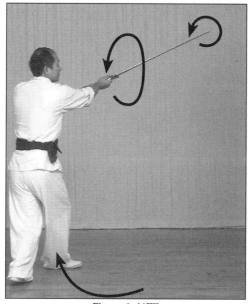

Figure 3-43W

Figure 3-43: White avoids Black's cut to his wrist by moving his sword handle counterclockwise, palm held downward. At the same time, White steps to the left (south) with the right leg across the front of his left leg. White cuts Black's wrist as he steps and lowers his hands.

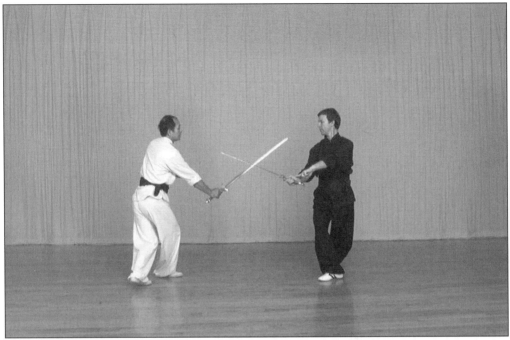

Figure 3-44

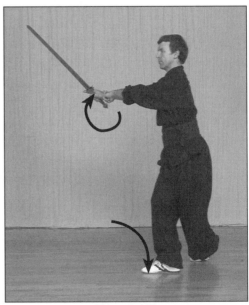

Figure 3-44B

Figure 3-44: Before White gets to cut Black, Black steps his right foot north into the crossed leg stance and circles his sword handle toward the north to avoid the cut, returning the left hand to the right wrist. For the next several forms the opponents' swords and sword arms circle around each other.

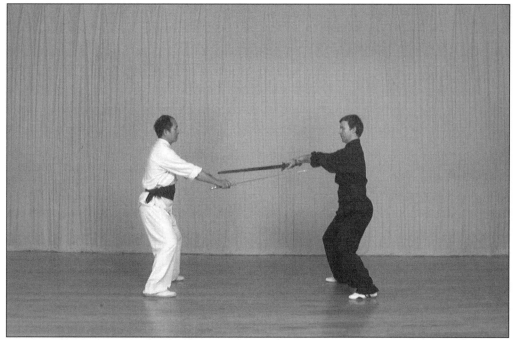

Figure 3-45

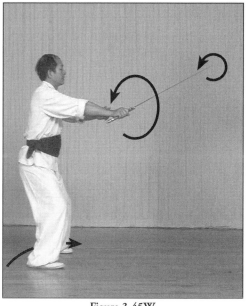

Figure 3-45W

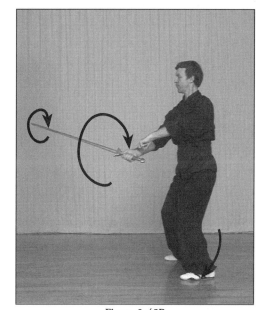

Figure 3-45B

Figure 3-45: White steps to the left with his left leg into the horse stance facing west and continues to circle his sword counterclockwise. Black also changes to the horse stance as he continues his clockwise circular cutting of White's wrist. White faces west, while Black faces east.

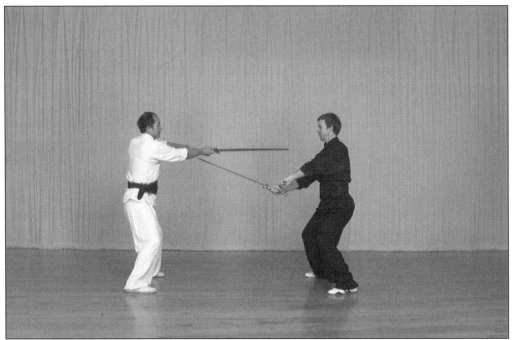

Figure 3-46

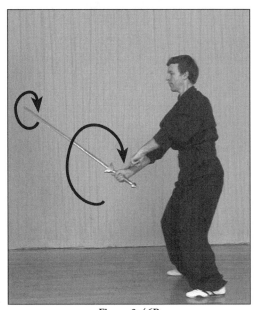

Figure 3-46B

Figures 3-46 to 3-48: Both White and Black continue circling each others' wrist, attempting to cut the other for two complete circles. Finally, Black gets to cover White's sword, allowing further action.

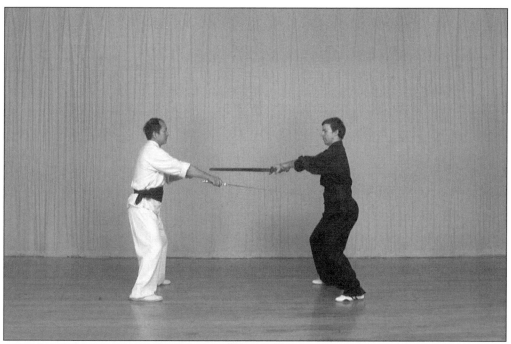

Figure 3-47

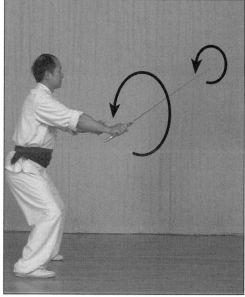

Figure 3-47W

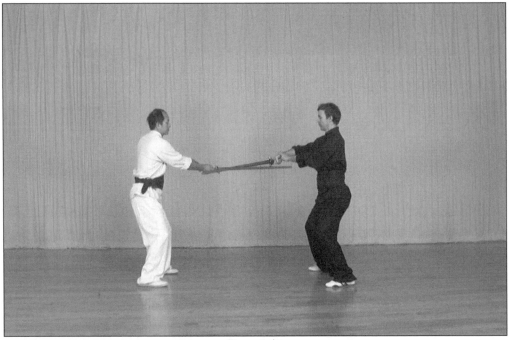

Figure 3-48

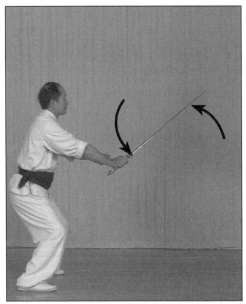

Figure 3-48W

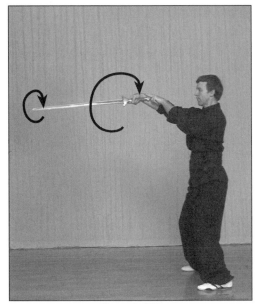

Figure 3-48B

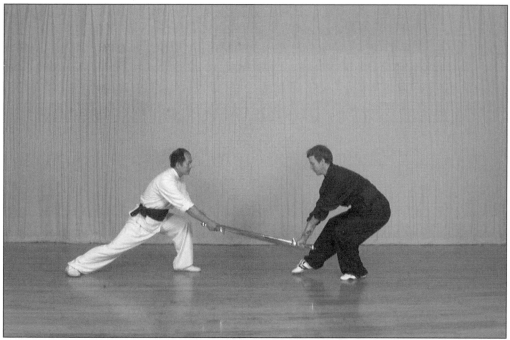

Figure 3-49

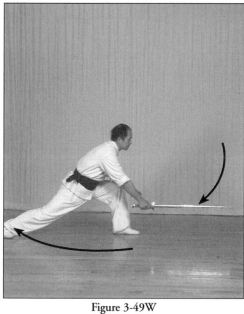

Figure 3-49W

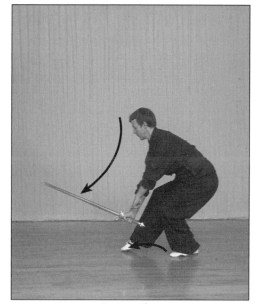

Figure 3-49B

Figure 3-49: When Black's sword is over White's, Black pushes White's sword down to the ground, as he bends low into the false stance. Feeling that his sword is trapped, White steps back with his right leg into the bow and arrow stance.

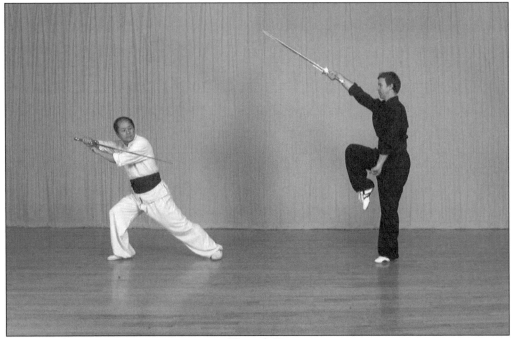

Figure 3-50

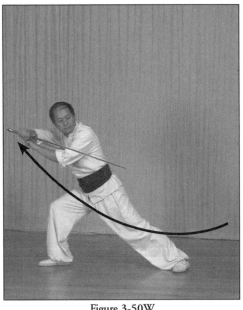

Figure 3-50W

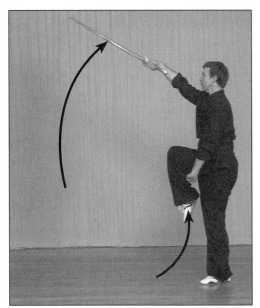

Figure 3-50B

Figure 3-50: White withdraws his sword from under Black's by pulling his arms back and shifting to the right into the bow and arrow stance. White's sword still points west toward Black, right palm down. As White slides away, Black stands upright raising his body and right leg to prepare for his next attack. Black's sword simply rises straight from the floor to the position shown as the left hand stays low

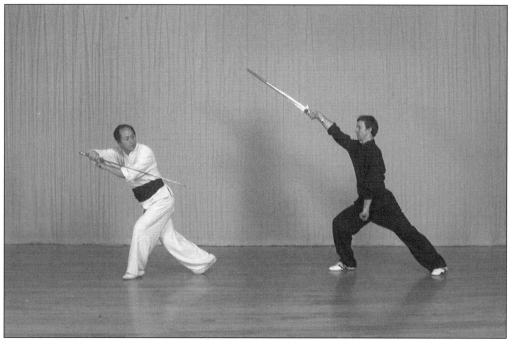

Figure 3-51

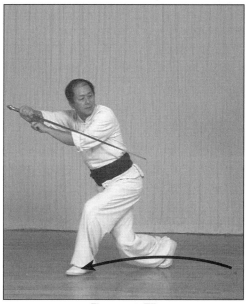
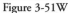

Figure 3-51W

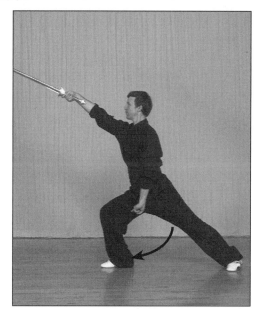

Figure 3-51B

in the secret sword position, pointing to the right in front of the groin.

Figure 3-51: Black begins his attack by stepping down into the bow and arrow stance with the right foot. White immediately starts walking away to the east as Black approaches, keeping the same hand positions, and stepping east with his leg. White continues to watch Black.

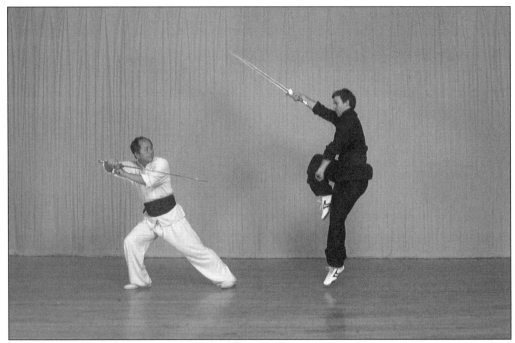

Figure 3-52

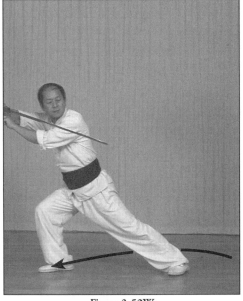

Figure 3-52W

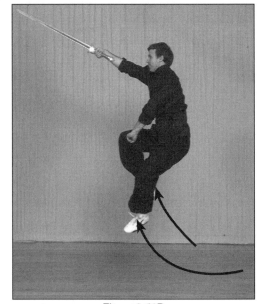

Figure 3-52B

Figure 3-52: To catch up with White, Black jumps up and toward White. White continues retreating by stepping back with his right foot. White ends up with his right leg forward on the second step in the bow and arrow stance. In solo practice, White should step four steps instead of two for withdrawing practice.

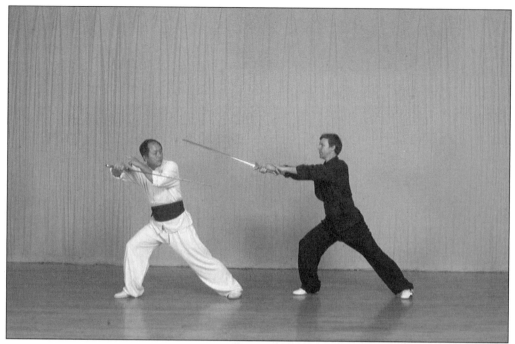

Figure 3-53

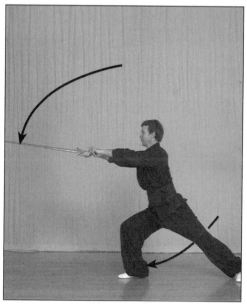

Figure 3-53B

Figure 3-53: Black lands on his left leg and steps toward White with his right into the bow and arrow stance as he chops down at White's head and touches his right wrist with his left fingers.

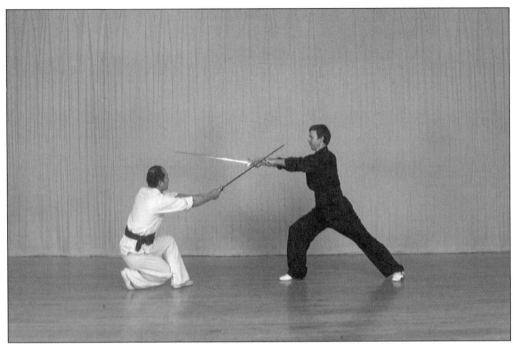

Figure 3-54

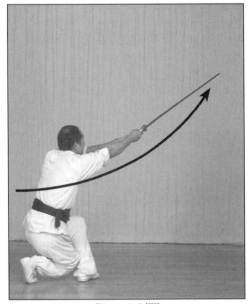

Figure 3-54W

Figure 3-54: As Black's chop approaches, White twists to the left into the crossed leg stance to face Black and thrusts his sword forward and upward to cut Black's wrist as Black's sword approaches.

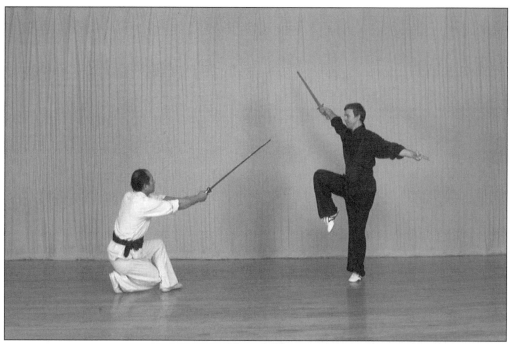

Figure 3-55

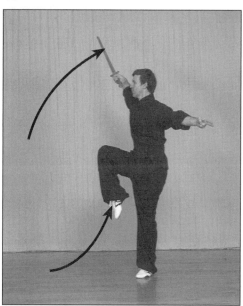

Figure 3-55B

Figure 3-55: Black, upon seeing White's attack, raises his right leg, while opening his arms to avoid White's attack.

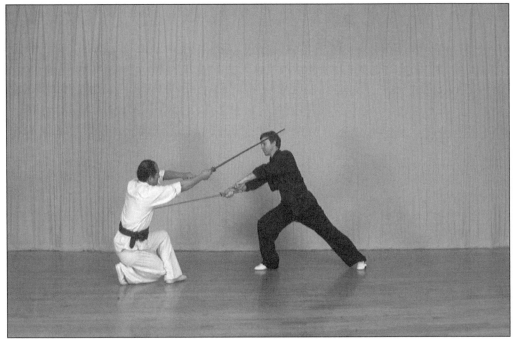

Figure 3-56

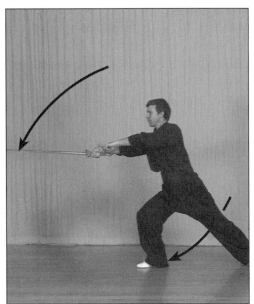

Figure 3-56B

Figure 3-56: Black then steps down slightly to the southeast and chops down diagonally at White's head.

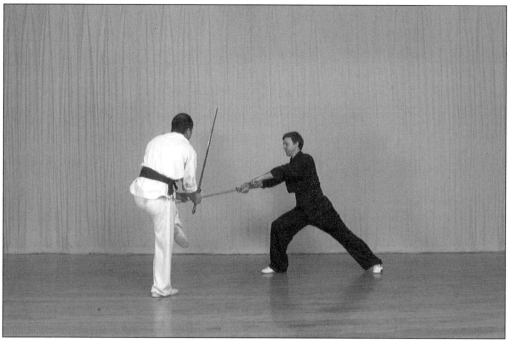

Figure 3-57

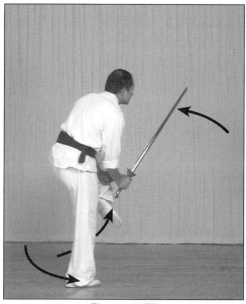

Figure 3-57W

Figure 3-57: White avoids this last attack by stepping his right foot to the northwest, and then raising the left foot. White drops his sword handle down to keep his sword in front of his opponent's.

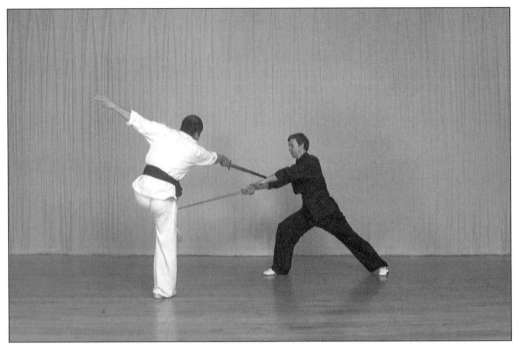

Figure 3-58

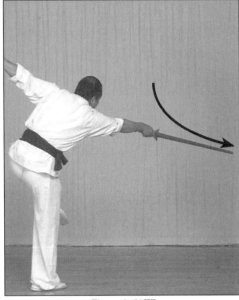

Figure 3-58W

Figure 3-58: White continues the motion and thrusts his sword forward to slice Black's wrist. White's left hand points in the opposite direction from his sword.

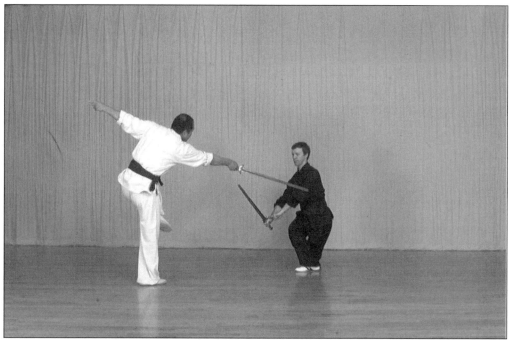

Figure 3-59

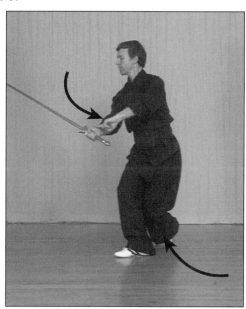

Figure 3-59B

Figure 3-59: Black avoids getting cut by simply moving his hands to the left and stepping with his left leg behind his right leg into the crossed leg stance.

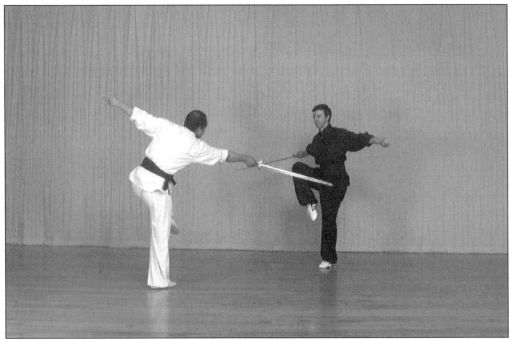

Figure 3-60

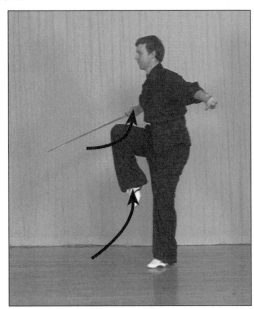

Figure 3-60B

Figure 3-60: Black continues this motion by lifting up his right leg and opening both hands as shown.

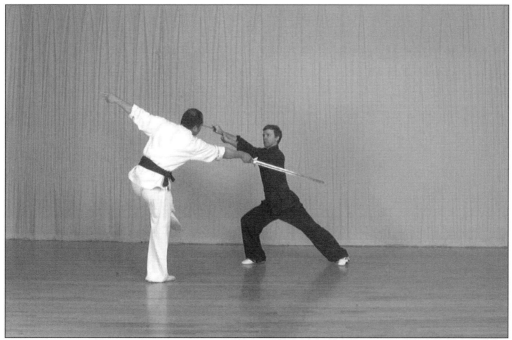

Figure 3-61

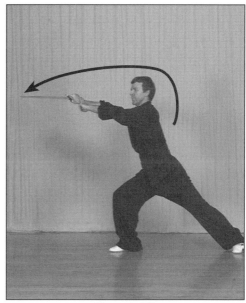

Figure 3-61B

Figure 3-61: Black continues this motion by stepping down with his leg into the bow and arrow stance and moving his sword upward to the right, keeping the blade horizontal, and stabbing White's face. This is the same as White's attack in Figure 3-41. White's sword is now to Black's left.

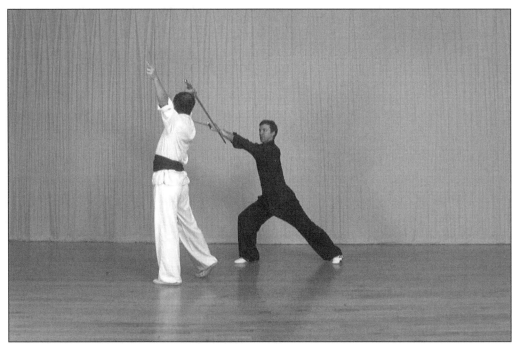

Figure 3-62

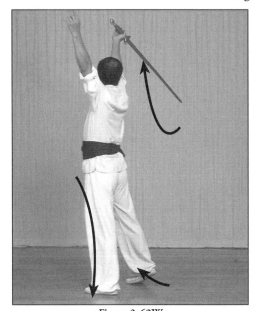

Figure 3-62W

Figure 3-62: As Black's sword approaches, White quickly steps down with the left leg to the north (White's sword is now pointing south), and turns his right wrist 180 degrees to the left, palm up, dropping the point of the sword to slice Black's wrist. White's right toes touch the ground.

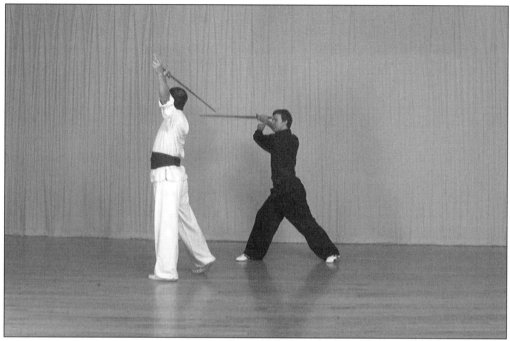

Figure 3-63

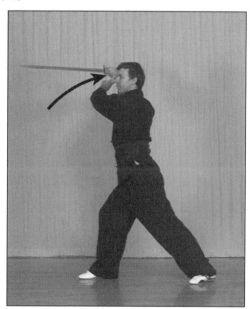

Figure 3-63B

Figure 3-63: Black avoids the attack by twisting his body to the right and withdrawing his sword.

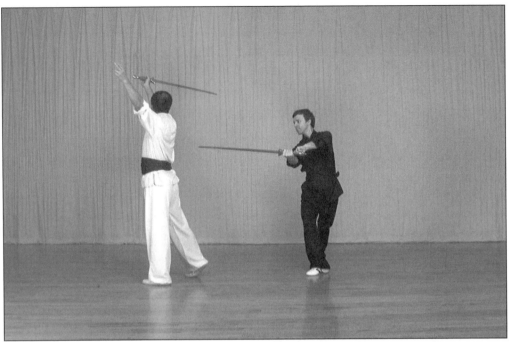

Figure 3-64

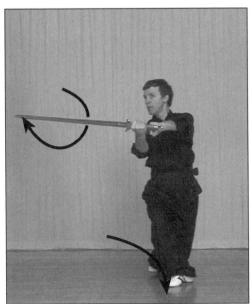

Figure 3-64B

Figure 3-64: Black continues this motion by shifting his weight to his left leg and then stepping to the north with his right leg into the crossed leg stance. As Black steps, he brings the sword hilt in toward his stomach and then to his left side, then thrusts his sword to White's back.

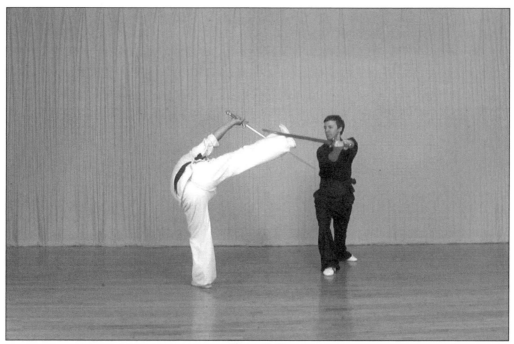

Figure 3-65

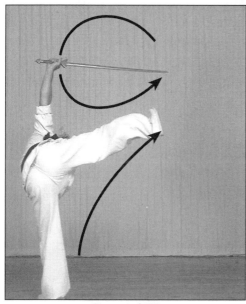

Figure 3-65W

Figure 3-65: As Black's sword approaches, White first lowers his entire upper body to a horizontal position, bringing his hands together at the chest. White continues by twisting his lowered body to the right and raising his right foot as shown to block the sword. At the same time, White's sword moves down to the left, then back up to cut Black's wrist.

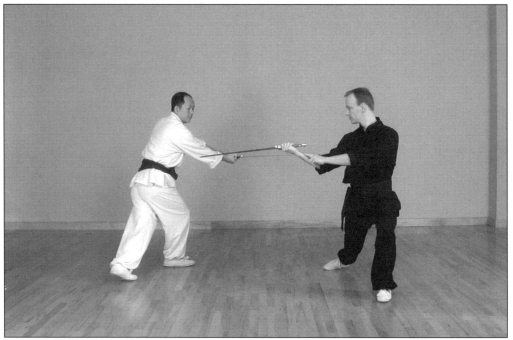

Figure 3-66

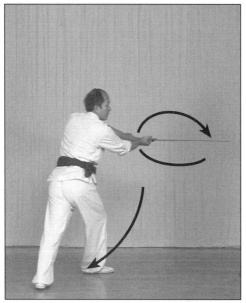

Figure 3-66W

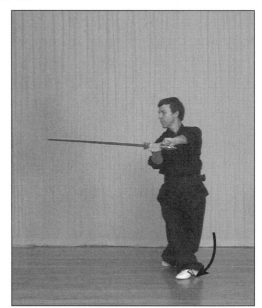

Figure 3-66B

Figure 3-66: Black avoids White's attack by merely stepping forward with his left leg into the bow and arrow stance, keeping the hand positions the same. As Black steps, White turns to the left and steps south with his right leg. At the same time he moves the sword in a clockwise circle and tries to stab Black with the same technique Black used in Figure 3-64.

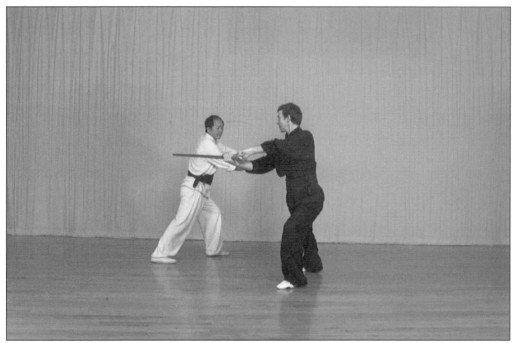

Figure 3-67

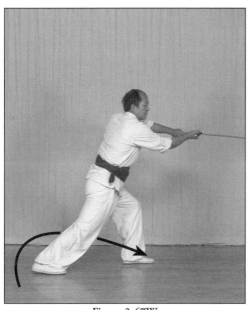

Figure 3-67W

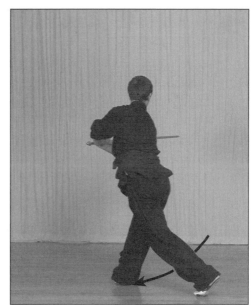

Figure 3-67B

Figure 3-67: Black continues this motion by stepping to the northeast around White with his right foot into the crossed leg stance as he begins to circle west at sword's length. White also continues his motion by stepping left leg forward into the bow and arrow stance.

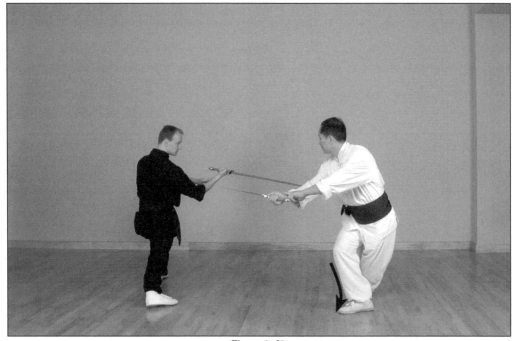

Figure 3-68

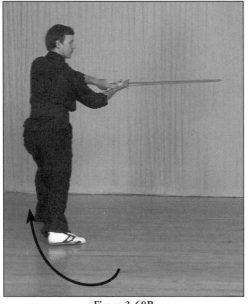

Figure 3-68B

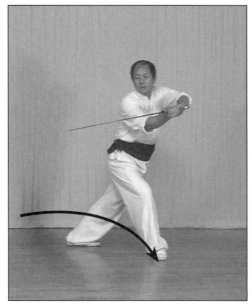

Figure 3-68W

Figure 3-68: Both White and Black continue circling each other as Black steps around to the side of White with the left foot into the bow and arrow stance as shown, now facing west. As Black steps, White also steps his forward with his right foot into the crossed leg stance now facing east.

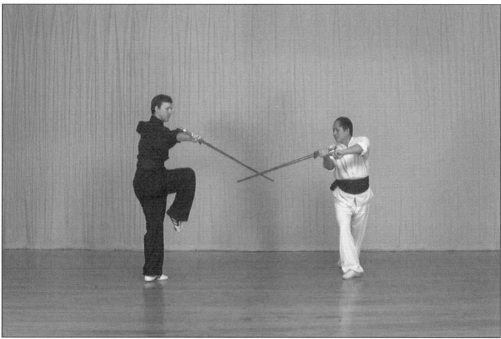

Figure 3-69

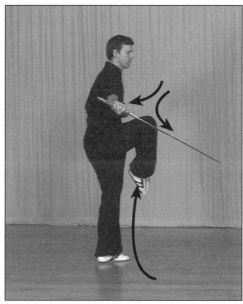

Figure 3-69B

Figure 3-69: Black twists his right wrist counterclockwise, turning his palm down and covers White's sword down and to his right (north) as Black also raises his right foot as shown. Black's left hand spreads to his left (south).

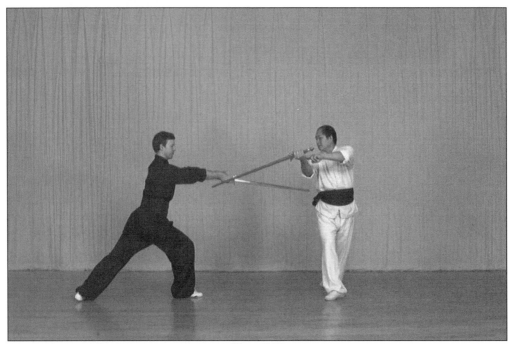

Figure 3-70

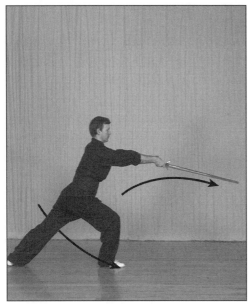

Figure 3-70B

Figure 3-70: Upon blocking White's sword to the side, Black steps forward into a bow and arrow stance and thrusts his sword toward White with his left fingers touching his right wrist.

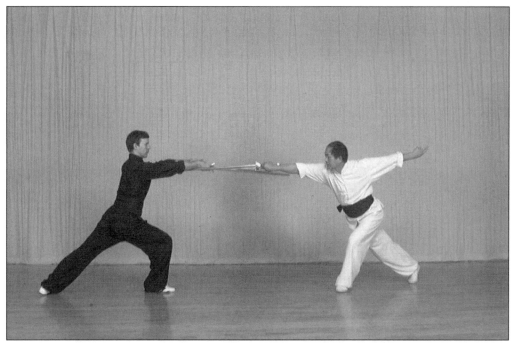

Figure 3-71

Figure 3-71: White avoids Black's attack by jumping with his left foot back (west), away from Black's sword. White lands by coming down first with his left foot as he twists his body to the right. When his left foot lands, his right foot stretches backward to the west and touches at the toes only. As he jumps, White's sword moves counterclockwise, the tip traveling up over his head, then

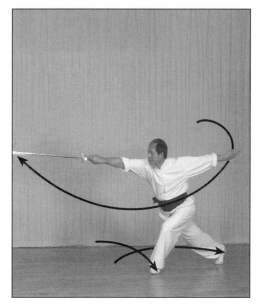

Figure 3-71W

back down and up to cut the underside of Black's wrist. White's palm now faces south. White's left palm also twists counterclockwise and faces south with the fingers pointing west. White is now facing east and Black west.

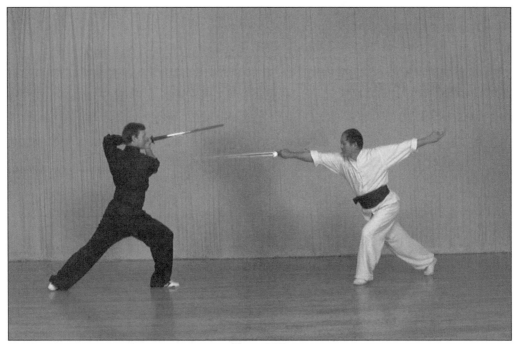

Figure 3-72

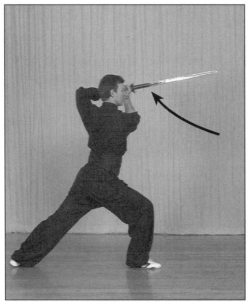

Figure 3-72B

Figure 3-72: Black avoids White's cut to his wrist by withdrawing his arms and sword to his left.

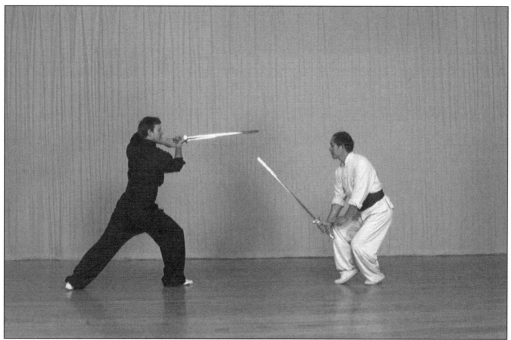

Figure 3-73

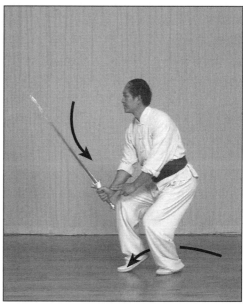

Figure 3-73B

Figure 3-73: Seeing Black withdraw, White advances by bringing his right leg forward into the false stance as he brings his hands together and lowers the sword hilt down beside his right knee.

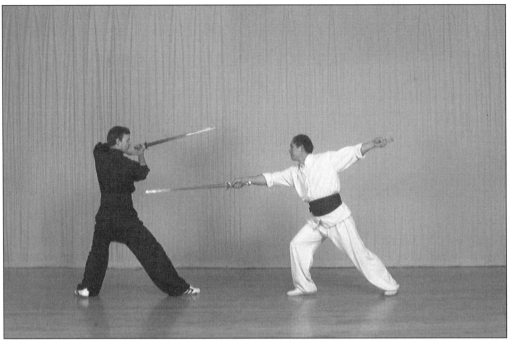

Figure 3-74

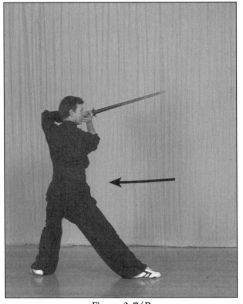

Figure 3-74B

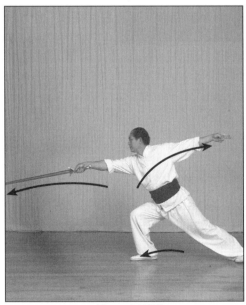

Figure 3-74W

Figure 3-74: White continues his advance by stepping forward with his right leg into the bow and arrow stance and thrusting his sword forward to Black's stomach with his left hand pointing backward. In order to avoid White's attack, Black sits back into the four-six stance.

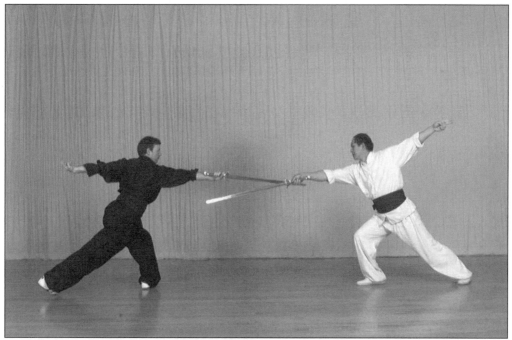

Figure 3-75

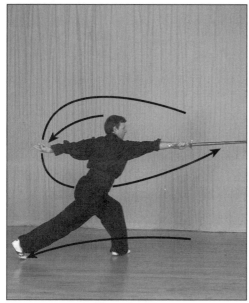

Figure 3-75B

Figure 3-75: As White's sword approaches, Black steps back with his right leg, touching only with the toes. As he steps back, Black turns his sword counterclockwise as the tip travels up, back (east), down, and then up at White's wrists. Black's wrist now faces north with the left hand pointing backward.

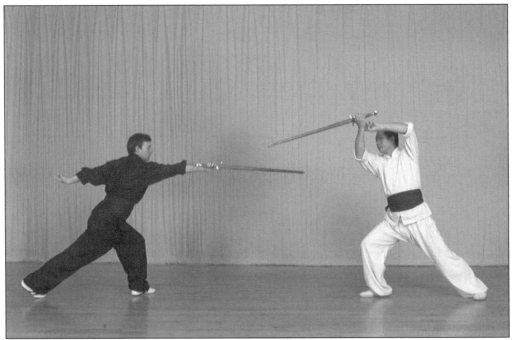

Figure 3-76

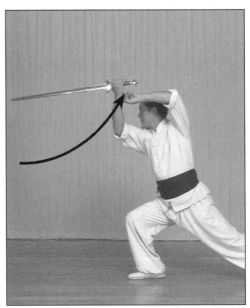

Figure 3-76W

Figure 3-76: White avoids Black's attack by simply withdrawing his sword back and to his left as Black did in Figure 3-72.

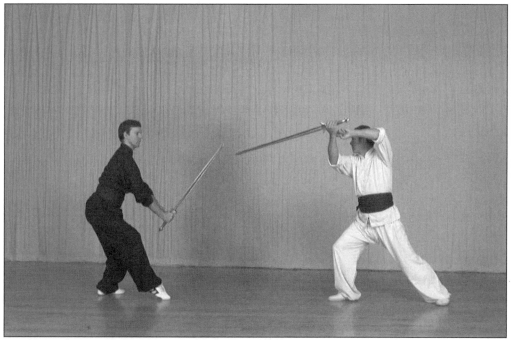

Figure 3-77

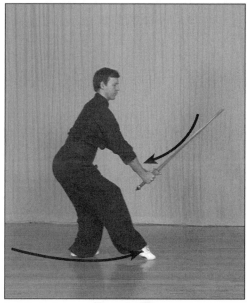

Figure 3-77B

Figure 3-77: Black now sees White's withdrawal and prepares his attack by stepping forward with his right foot into the false stance as White did in Figure 3-73. Black moves his sword and arms to the position shown.

121

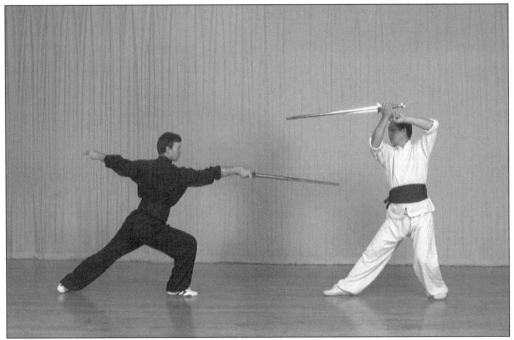

Figure 3-78

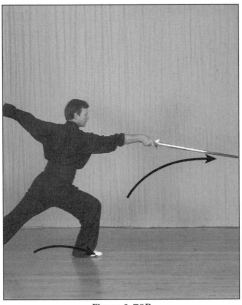
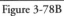

Figure 3-78B

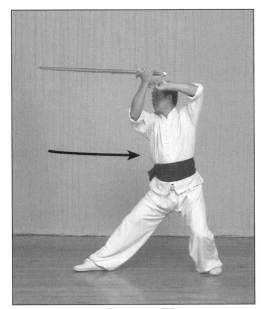

Figure 3-78W

Figure 3-78: Black continues his motion by thrusting forward with his sword as he steps forward with his right foot into the bow and arrow stance. In order to avoid Black's attack, White sits back into the four-six stance.

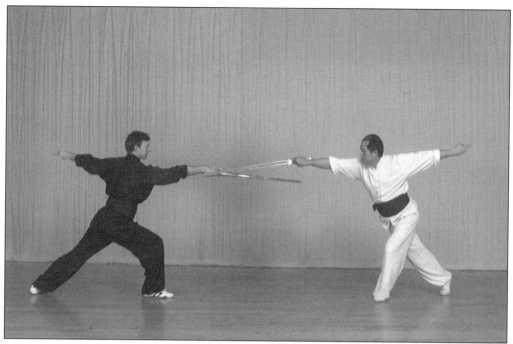

Figure 3-79

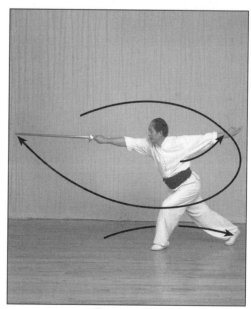

Figure 3-79W

Figure 3-79: As Black's sword approaches, White steps back with his right leg, touching only with the toes. As he steps back, White turns his sword counterclockwise as the tip travels up, back, down, and then up at Black's wrists. White's left hand points backward.

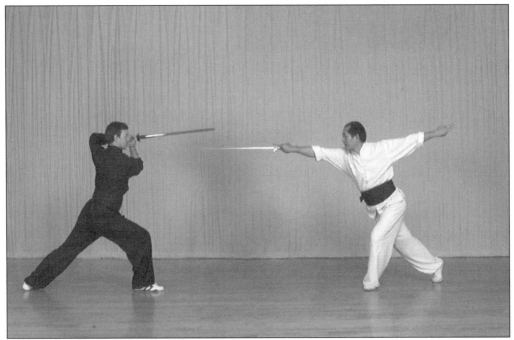

Figure 3-80

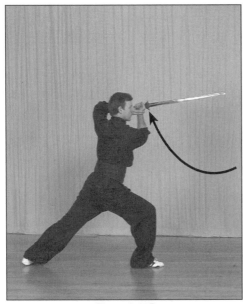

Figure 3-80B

Figures 3-80 to 3-88: Repeat from Figures 3-72 to 3-79 then Figure 3-72. See instructions for these figures.

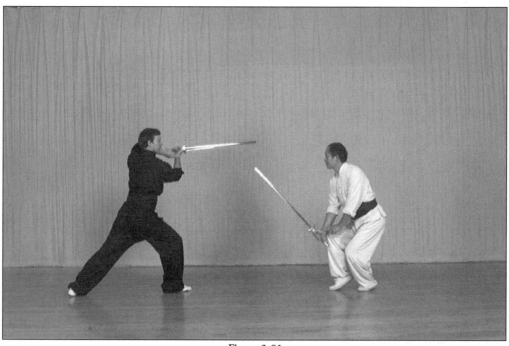

Figure 3-81

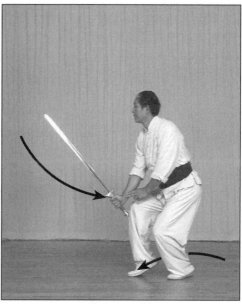

Figure 3-81W

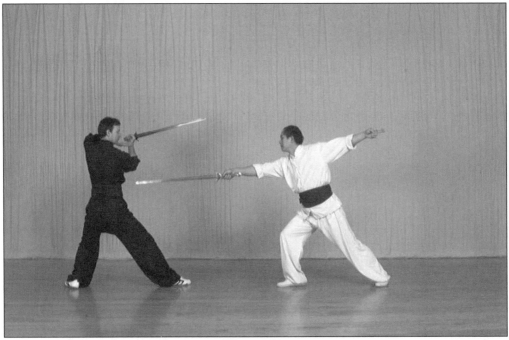

Figure 3-82

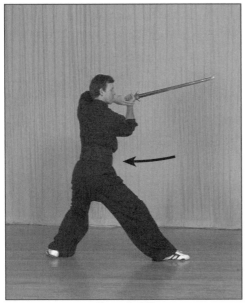

Figure 3-82B

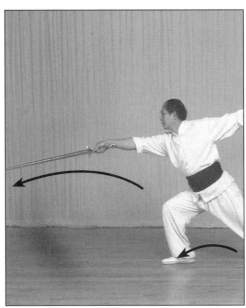

Figure 3-82W

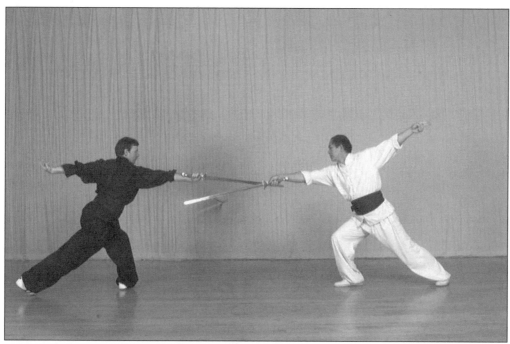

Figure 3-83

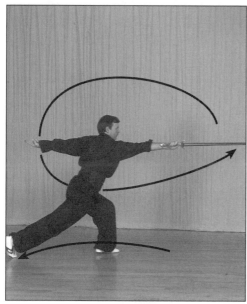

Figure 3-83B

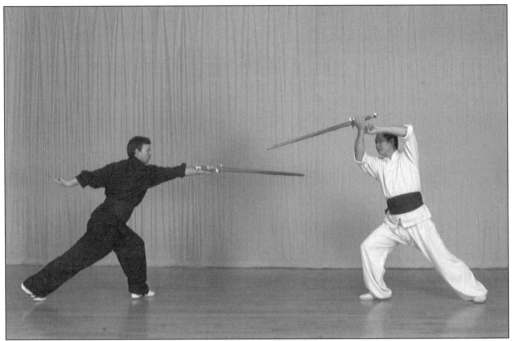

Figure 3-84

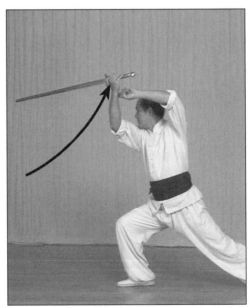

Figure 3-84W

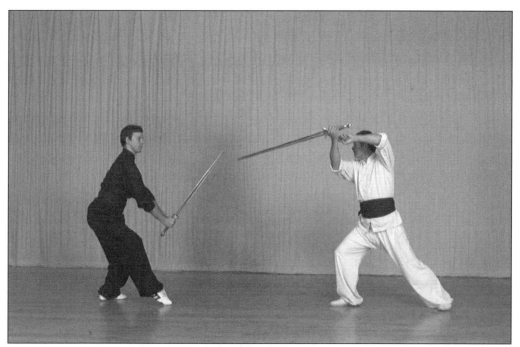

Figure 3-85

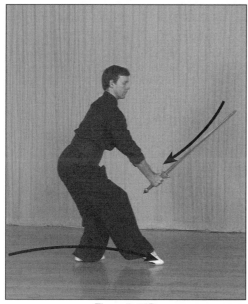

Figure 3-85B

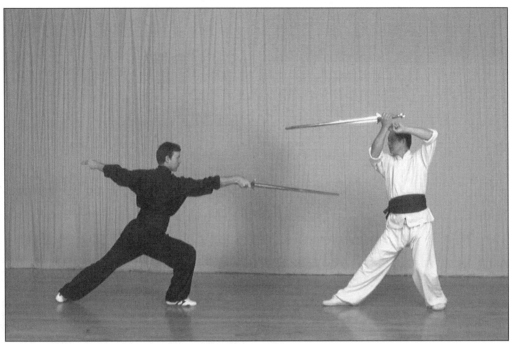

Figure 3-86

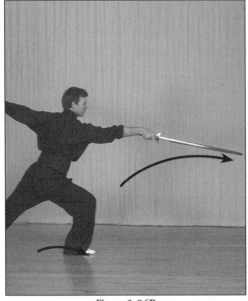

Figure 3-86B

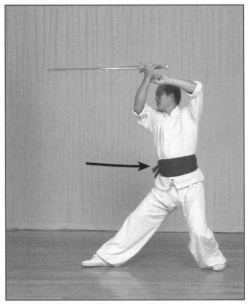

Figure 3-86W

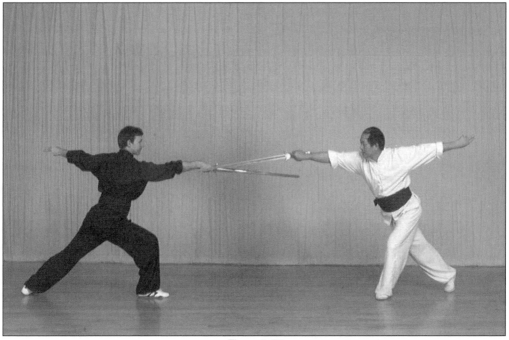

Figure 3-87

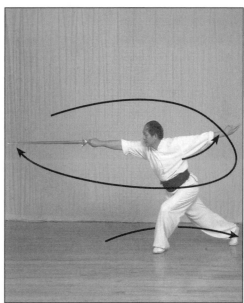

Figure 3-87W

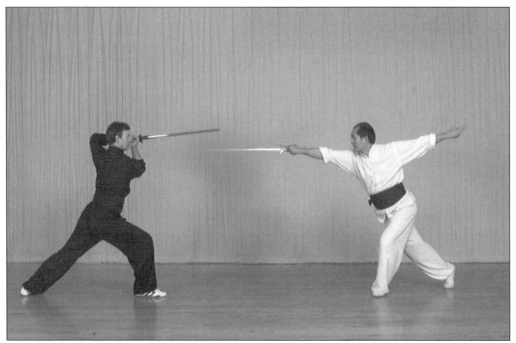

Figure 3-88

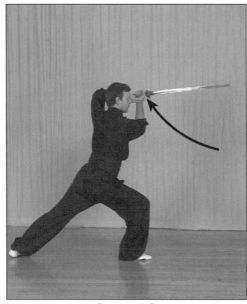

Figure 3-88B

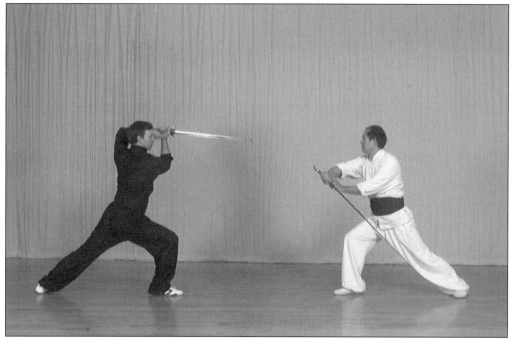

Figure 3-89

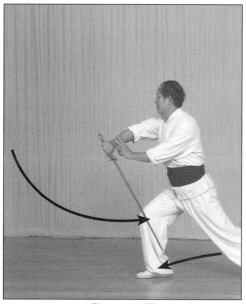

Figure 3-89W

Figure 3-89: This time when Black withdraws, White steps forward with his right leg into the bow and arrow stance as he lowers the tip of his sword and brings his hands together as shown.

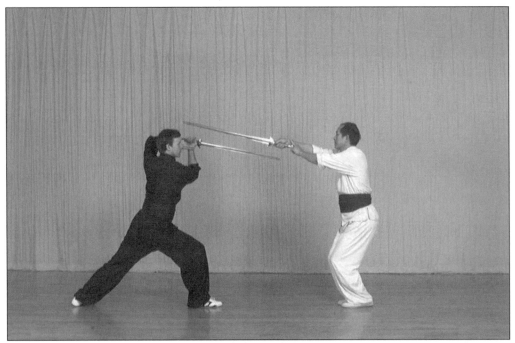

Figure 3-90

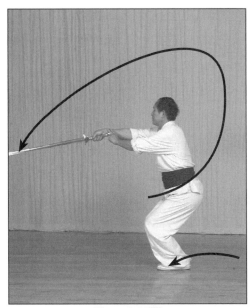

Figure 3-90W

Figure 3-90: White continues the circle with his sword up to face east and continues to rotate his wrist counterclockwise. The sword tip moves higher than his head. As the sword blade goes down to cut Black's head, White moves his left foot up beside his right as shown.

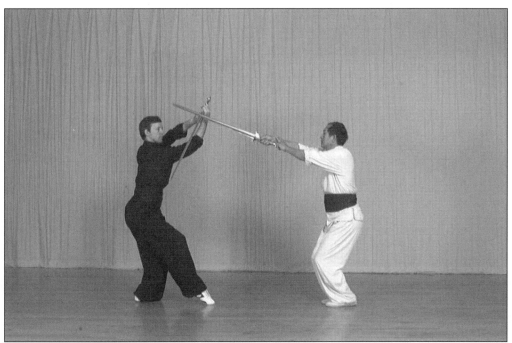

Figure 3-91

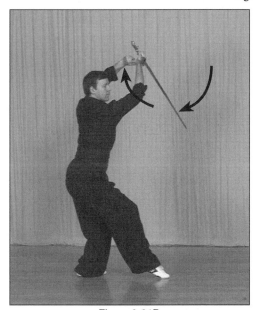

Figure 3-91B

Figure 3-91: As White's sword approaches, Black moves his right foot back into the false stance with the right leg forward. At the same time Black swings his arms to his left across his chest, keeping essentially the same form, but raising the handle slightly as shown to guide White's sword down and to his right side. Black's palms are held upward.

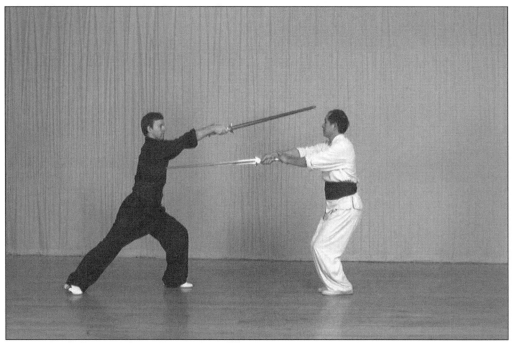

Figure 3-92

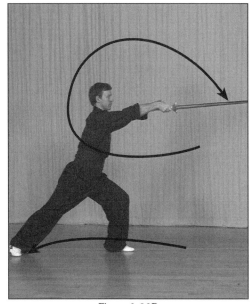

Figure 3-92B

Figure 3-92: As White's sword slides down and to the side, Black steps back with his right leg into the bow and arrow stance, left leg forward. At the same time, he drops the point of his sword and then rotates his right wrist counterclockwise, causing the tip of the sword to travel in a complete vertical circle, resulting in chopping down at White's head as shown. (Note: The arms stay relatively still because the turn-

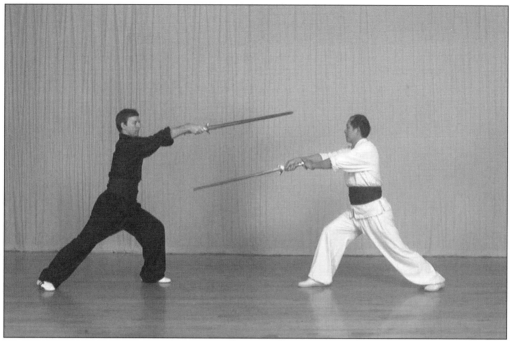

Figure 3-93

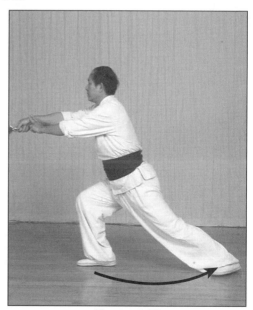

Figure 3-93W

ing of the wrist is used to slide Black's sword away from White's sword and to attack over the top.) Black's right wrist faces to his left (south).

Figure 3-93: White avoids Black's attack by merely stepping back with his left leg into the bow and arrow stance.

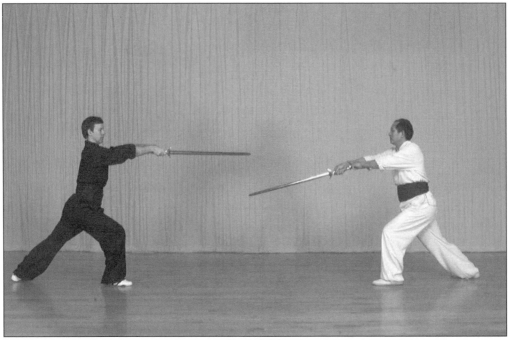

Figure 3-94

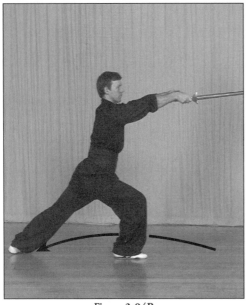

Figure 3-94B

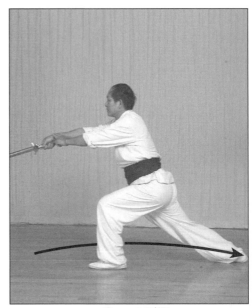

Figure 3-94W

Figure 3-94: Just after White steps back, Black also steps back with the left leg into the bow and arrow stance. At the same time White steps back with his right leg into the bow and arrow stance.

Figure 3-95: White continues his backward motion by stepping back with his left

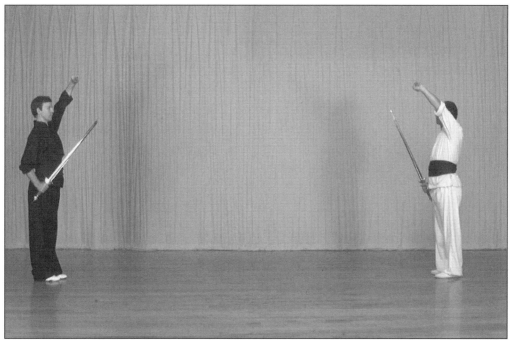

Figure 3-95

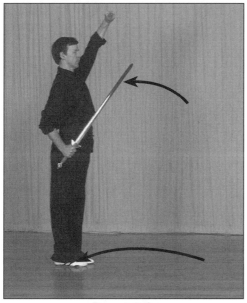

Figure 3-95B

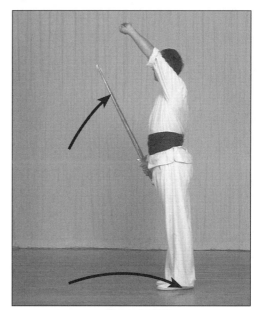

Figure 3-95W

foot beside his right and standing upright. At the same time, he drops his sword handle down and raises the tip as shown. White's left hand rises above his head, pointing to the right. Black also continues his backward motion by stepping back with his right foot beside the right and standing upright in the same form as White.

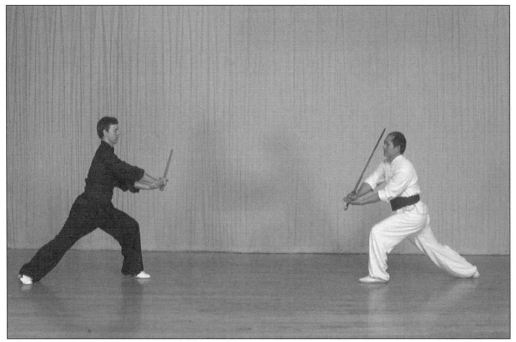

Figure 3-96

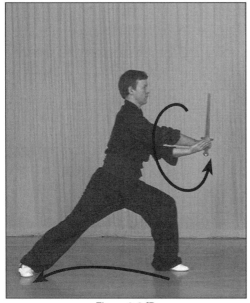

Figure 3-96B

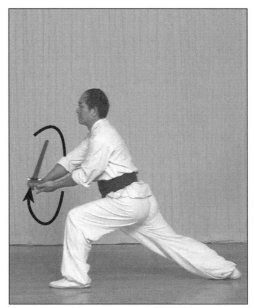

Figure 3-96W

Figures 3-96 and 3-97: Both White and Black step back with their right legs into the bow and arrow stance. At the same time they bring their left hand up in front of the chest, palm up, and the right hand places the handle of the sword beside the left

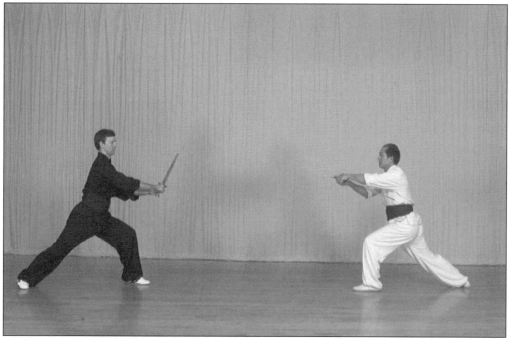

Figure 3-97

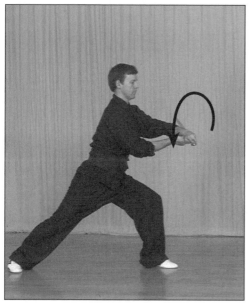

Figure 3-97B

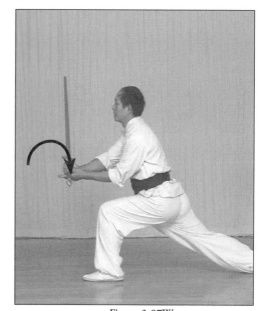

Figure 3-97W

hand. Both White and Black then continue the same motion by grasping the sword with the left hand and turning the left wrist clockwise so that the sword makes a full circle in front of the body.

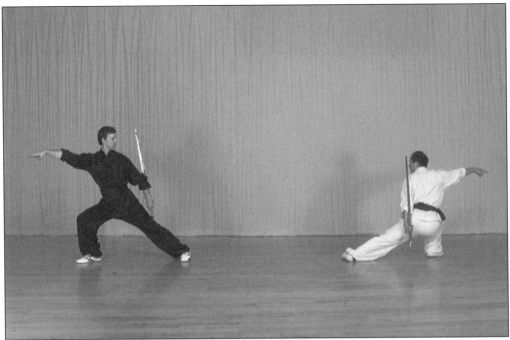

Figure 3-98

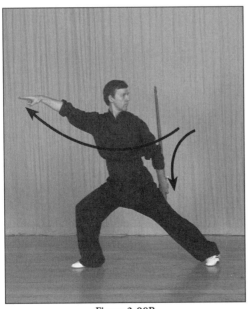

Figure 3-98B

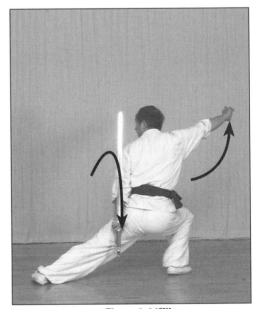

Figure 3-98W

Figure 3-98: As both partners' left hands begin to rotate, the right hands, held in the secret sword position, move next to the body, under the left armpit, palm up, then stretch to the right with palm downward. The left hands' fingers now point down with the left wrist facing backward. White and Black each twist their bodies to the right into the taming the tiger stance.

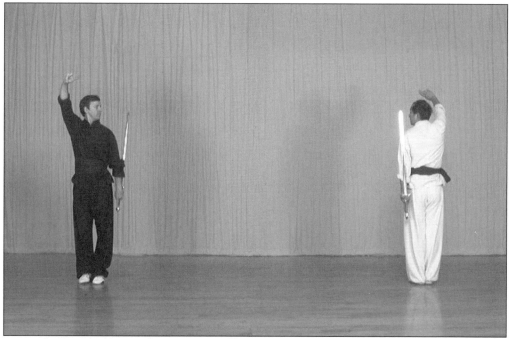

Figure 3-99

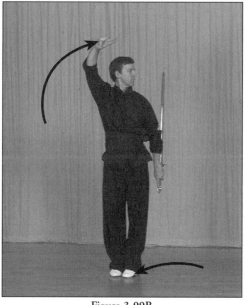

Figure 3-99B

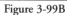

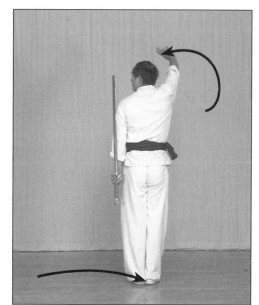

Figure 3-99W

Figure 3-99: White and Black each stand upright by placing the left foot up next to the right, and moving the right hand up and back into the position as shown. Each looks to the left with the right hand pointing to the left, palm outward. White faces south, Black north. For solo practice, the head looks forward.

CHAPTER 4

Kun Wu Jian

崑峿劍

4-1. INTRODUCTION

Kun Wu is the name of a mountain in southwest An Qiu Xian in Shandong Province (山東、安秋縣). It is also the name of swords produced from the high quality ore mined from this mountain. The sequence may have originated there as well, although the first historical reference occurs during the Qing Dynasty (1644-1911 A.D., 清朝), when Li, Yu-Xiang (李玉祥) was teaching it in Cang Xian, Hebei Province (河北、滄縣).

The sequence is more advanced than San Cai Jian, although the techniques in it are still basic. It should be learned after the San Cai Jian to improve sword technique and to gain further understanding of sword applications. In the illustrations the person in the white shirt demonstrates the solo form, while the person in the black shirt acts as the attacker in the application of the forms. The first level solution of every technique will be given. In the description of the moves, the direction originally faced is considered north.

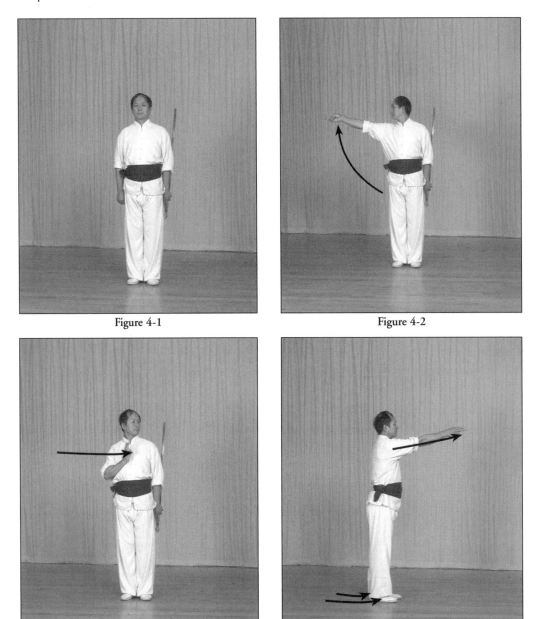

Figure 4-1

Figure 4-2

Figure 4-3

Figure 4-4

4-2. KUN WU JIAN

Figure 4-1: Stand upright facing north holding the sword with the left hand, palms facing south.

Figures 4-2 to 4-4: Look to the right (east) as the right hand rises to a horizontal position in the secret sword form. The right palm faces north. Bring the right hand

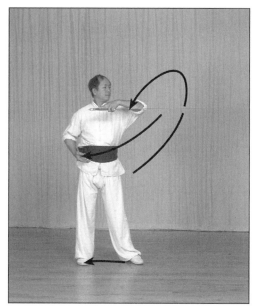

Figure 4-5

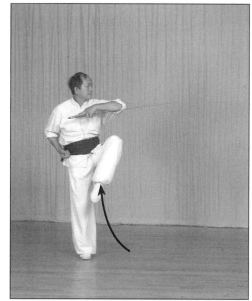

Figure 4-6

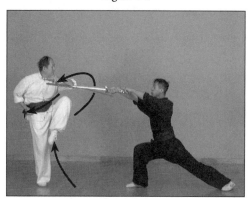

Figure 4-6A

to the chest with first and second fingers still extended, as the head turns and faces west. Turn and step to the left (west) as the right hand moves from the chest and points forward (west). As the right hand is extended, move the right leg forward beside the left as shown in Figure 4.

Figures 4-5 to 4-7: Move the right leg back as the right hand moves to the waist, palm up, and the left arm (holding the sword) moves up in front of the chest. With the same motion, the left arm and the sword continue to the right side of the body, palm down, as the left leg is raised, with the knee facing west. Immediately after the leg is raised, swing the right hand out from the body, then back in to meet the sword handle. The sword and body both face west now.

Figure 4-6A: Black attacks White, and White blocks with his leg raised for a possible kick.

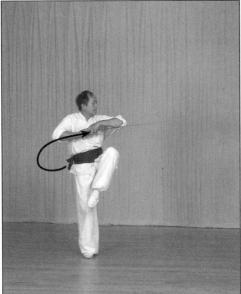

Figure 4-7

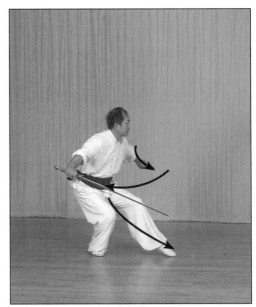

Figure 4-8

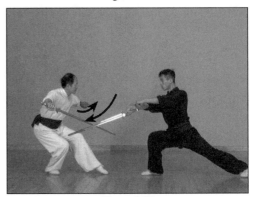

Figure 4-8A

Figure 4-8: Grasp the sword with the right hand and move both arms down, palms down, and step forward with the left leg into the false stance, with the left hand held in the secret sword position.

Figure 4-8A: Black attacks White, and White blocks as shown.

Figure 4-9: Step forward (west) with the left leg as both hands come together at the chest. The motion continues forward as you step with the right leg behind the left into the crossed leg stance (west). At the same time, thrust both arms forward (west) with the extended fingers of the left hand resting on the right wrist.

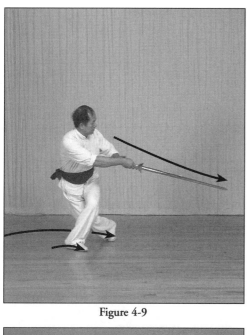

Figure 4-9

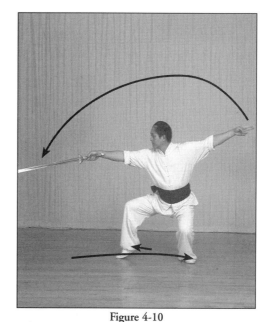

Figure 4-10

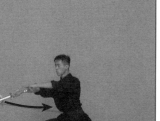

Figure 4-9A

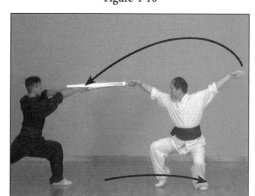

Figure 4-10A

Figure 4-9A: After blocking in Figure 4-8A, White steps toward Black and attacks the now open midsection.

Figure 4-10: Step backward (west) with the left leg as the body turns clockwise 180 degrees with the right leg forward in the false stance facing east. As the body turns, the sword moves over the head in the vertical plane from west to east to the position shown. At the same time point west and slightly up with the left hand.

Figure 4-10A: White steps backward with the left leg to avoid Black's attack from the back and at the same time chops down at Black's wrist as White's outstretched arms and body position keep him from danger.

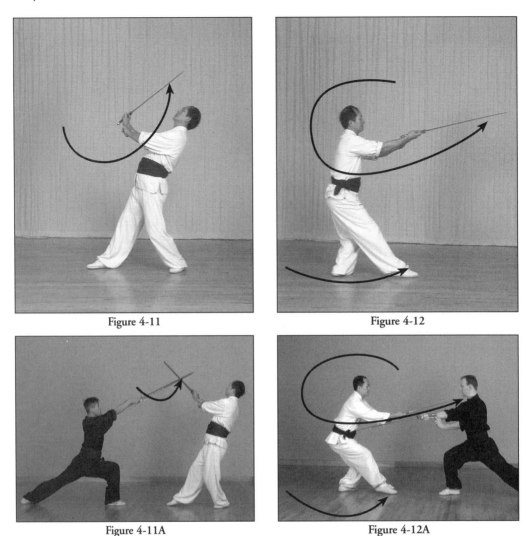

Figure 4-11

Figure 4-12

Figure 4-11A

Figure 4-12A

Figure 4-11: Touch the right wrist with the left fingers. Lean far back while making a clockwise circle with the sword in front of and above the body, right palm facing away from the body.

Figure 4-11A: White blocks Black's strike to the face.

Figure 4-12: As the circle is half completed, turn the body left 180 degrees to face west and step forward with the right leg into the false stance. The sword points forward (west), right palm facing up. The sword has moved through one and one half circles.

Figure 4-12A: After blocking in Figure 4-11A, White attacks Black's neck by following Black's sword inward. In the application, White does not turn the body 180 degrees.

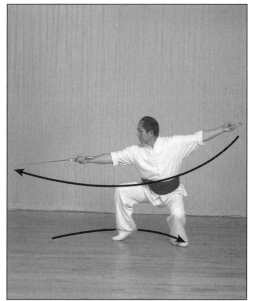

Figure 4-13

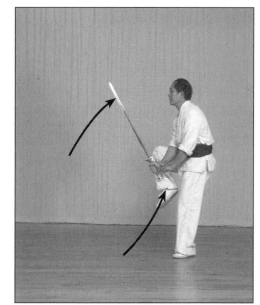

Figure 4-14

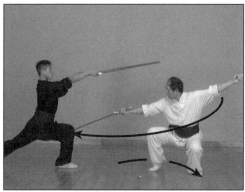

Figure 4-13A

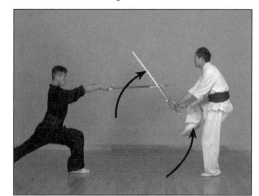

Figure 4-14A

Figure 4-13: Step down with the right foot and then step forward to the west with the left leg. As you step forward with the left leg, turn the body clockwise 180 degrees into the false stance with the right leg forward (east). Also, as the body turns, the left hand remains pointing west while the sword moves horizontally with the body into the position shown facing east. The right palm faces upward.

Figure 4-13A: White avoids Black's attack from the rear by moving low into the false stance and attacking Black's legs.

Figure 4-14: Move the sword in toward the body as the right leg rises into the golden rooster stands on one leg stance, while touching the left fingers to the right wrist. The right palm faces north.

Figure 4-14A: By moving the sword back toward the body, White guides Black's sword to the side.

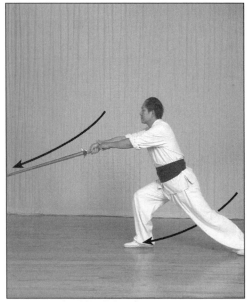

Figure 4-15

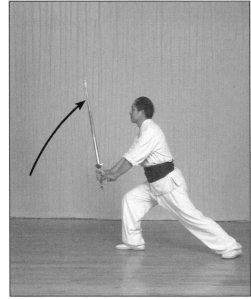

Figure 4-16

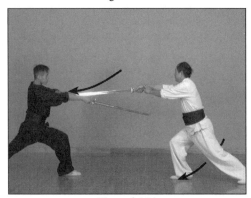

Figure 4-15A

Figure 4-15: Step down with the right leg into the bow and arrow stance and thrust the sword forward.

Figure 4-15A: After blocking in Figure 4-14A, White attacks Black's forearm.

Figure 4-16: Move the sword back to the body as in Figure 4-14, but remain in the bow and arrow stance with the right leg forward.

Figure 4-17: After the previous block, step forward with the left leg into the bow and arrow stance and thrust the sword forward.

Figure 4-18: While in the same stance, move the sword in toward the body and block again as in Figure 4-16.

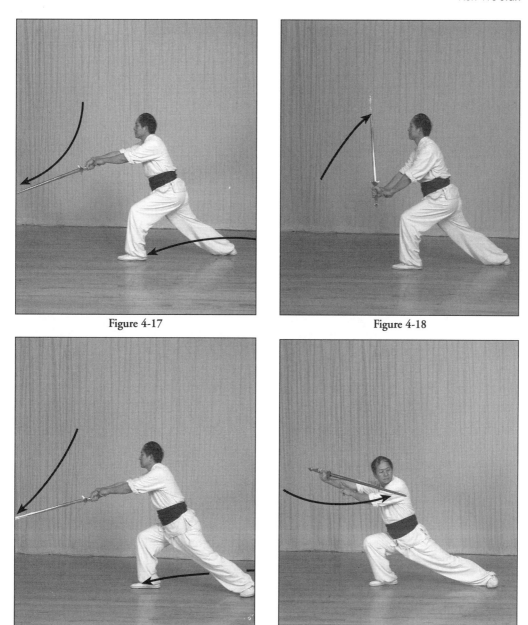

Figure 4-17

Figure 4-18

Figure 4-19

Figure 4-20

Figure 4-19: Step forward with the right leg into the bow and arrow stance and thrust the sword forward. The left fingers remain on the right wrist. Figures 4-15 to 4-19 are executed in three quick steps, the body staying low.

Figure 4-20: Turn the body 90 degrees counterclockwise into the taming the tiger stance and point the sword west while keeping the right arm extended and pointing east, and look to the west.

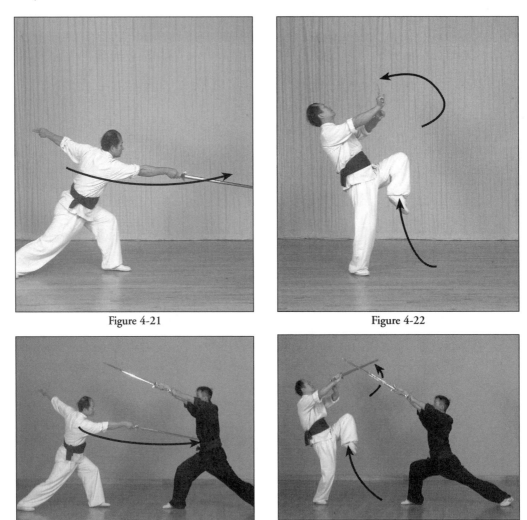

Figure 4-21

Figure 4-22

Figure 4-21A

Figure 4-22A

Figure 4-21: Move the stance forward into the bow and arrow stance with the left leg forward, and thrust the sword forward (west) as the left hand swings counter-clockwise with the body and points east.

Figure 4-21A: White attacks Black's midsection.

Figures 4-22 and 4-23: Raise the left leg up into the golden rooster stands on one leg stance as the left hand returns to the right wrist. Also, as the leg is raised, repeat the block in Figure 4-11, leaning backward and moving the sword in a clockwise cir-cle at approximately a 45 degree angle to the rear. End up as shown in Figure 4-23 with the right palm facing upward.

Figures 4-22A and 4-23A: White blocks Black's attack and then attacks Black's neck by following Black's sword back inward.

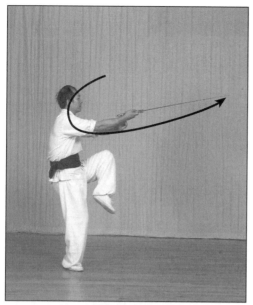

Figure 4-23

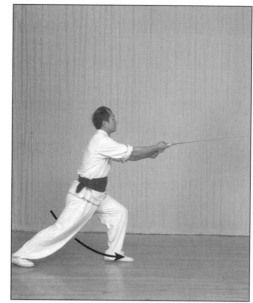

Figure 4-24

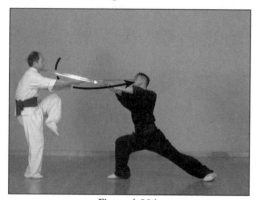

Figure 4-23A

Figure 4-24: Step forward with the left leg into the bow and arrow stance while moving the right hand in small, counterclockwise circular motions.

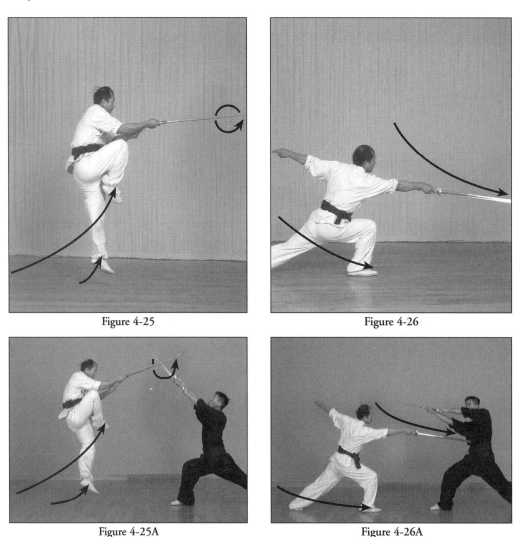

Figure 4-25

Figure 4-26

Figure 4-25A

Figure 4-26A

Figures 4-25 and 4-26: Continue the forward motion and jump off the left leg, bringing the right knee up high and end up with the right leg forward in the bow and arrow stance. As the right leg comes down into the bow and arrow stance, thrust the sword forward while pointing the left hand behind to the east. Continue the small and continuous counterclockwise motion of the wrist three times before the thrust in Figure 4-26.

Figure 4-25A: The counterclockwise motion blocks Black's sword to the side to allow for the thrust forward.

Figure 4-26A: White attacks Black's midsection.

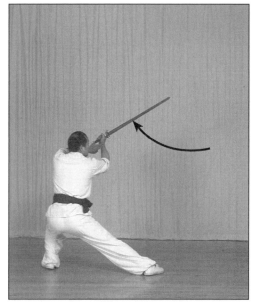

Figure 4-27

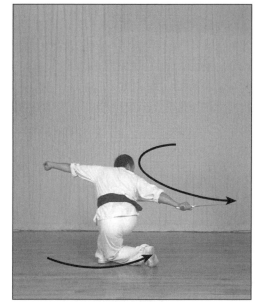

Figure 4-28

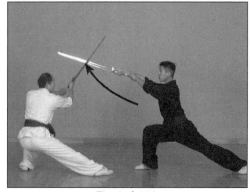

Figure 4-27A

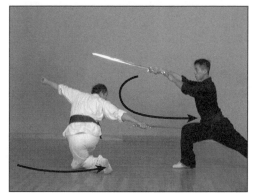

Figure 4-28A

Figure 4-27: Shift the weight to the left leg into the taming the tiger stance. At the same time, touch the right wrist with the left fingers and raise both arms.

Figure 4-27A: White shifts his weight back and the sword to the side to guide Black's sword away.

Figure 4-28: Move the left foot behind and to the west of the right foot into the crossed leg stance. At the same time, extend the left arm to the east while cutting down and forward at a 45 degree angle with the sword, palm held downward.

Figure 4-28A: After the block in Figure 4-27A, White steps in and attacks Black's leg.

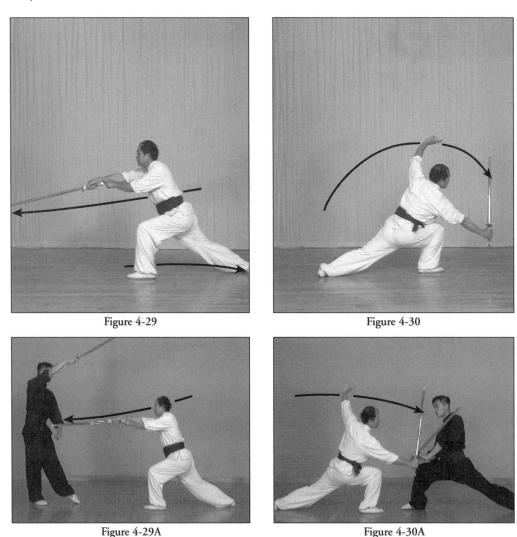

Figure 4-29

Figure 4-30

Figure 4-29A

Figure 4-30A

Figure 4-29: Move the right leg back (west) into the bow and arrow stance facing east with the left leg forward. At the same time touch the right wrist with the left fingers and thrust the sword forward to the east slightly downward.

Figure 4-29A: White attacks Black's midsection.

Figure 4-30: Shift to the bow and arrow stance in the other direction (west) by turning to the right. At the same time keep the right arm straight and move the sword in a clockwise motion to a vertical position. This is a very low bow and arrow stance, facing west.

Figure 4-30A: White presses Black's sword to stop Black's attack.

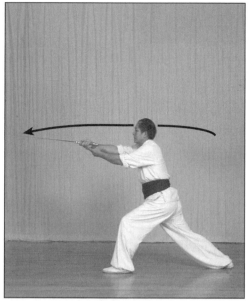

Figure 4-31

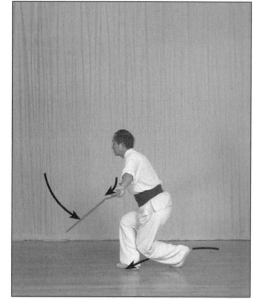

Figure 4-32

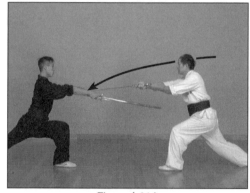

Figure 4-31A

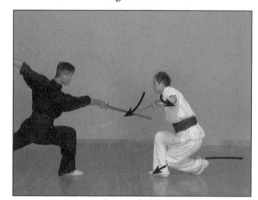

Figure 4-32A

Figure 4-31: Shift the same stance back to the east by turning to the left. This time, the sword cuts in a horizontal plane in the same direction. Return the left fingers to the right wrist.

Figure 4-31A: White cuts Black's wrist or neck.

Figure 4-32: Step forward to the east with the right leg into the unicorn stance while blocking down and out as in Figure 4-8.

Figure 4-32A: White guides Black's attack to the side.

Figure 4-33: Step forward with the left leg while bringing the two hands together down and in front of the body but keeping both arms straight. Continue the motion forward by stepping with the right foot next to the left and stand up straight.

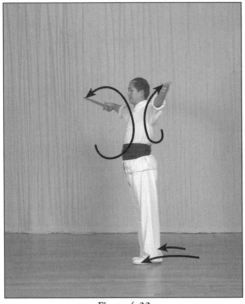

Figure 4-33

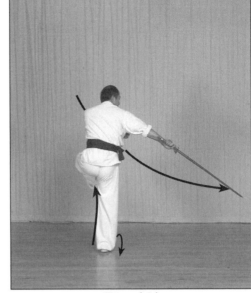

Figure 4-34

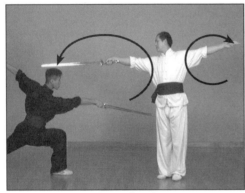

Figure 4-33A

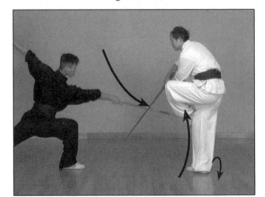

Figure 4-34A

At the same time this motion occurs, continue the motion of the arms in a circular and vertical direction (right arm clockwise, left arm counterclockwise), crossing at the chest, stretching out above the head and ending the circle as shown, with the palms facing forward (body faces east throughout).

Figure 4-33A: After blocking in Figure 4-32A, White attacks Black's head with a downward chopping motion.

Figure 4-34: Raise the right foot slightly off the floor and stomp down with it while hopping up with the left knee. Turn the body 45 degrees to the right as this hop occurs while bringing the left fingers to the right wrist and moving the sword straight down from the position of Figure 4-33 to the position shown.

Figure 4-34A: White guides Black's sword away with a downward motion of his sword.

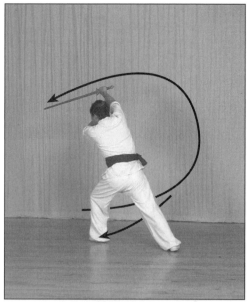

Figure 4-35

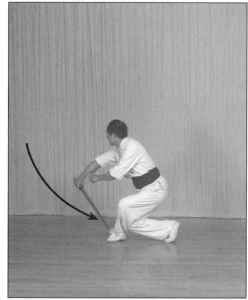

Figure 4-36

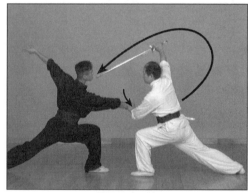

Figure 4-35A

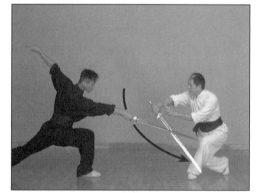

Figure 4-36A

Figure 4-35: Continue this counterclockwise motion with the sword down, behind, and then over the head to the position shown. The left hand leaves the right wrist briefly, then joins it again at the position shown. At the same time as the sword thrusts forward, step with the left leg into the bow and arrow stance.

Figure 4-35A: After blocking in Figure 4-34A, White steps in beside Black's sword and continues in the same motion to attack Black's throat.

Figure 4-36: Twist the body to the left into the crossed leg stance while moving the sword in a circular motion down and to the left side with the sword pointing to the rear (northwest).

Figure 4-36A: White guides Black's sword to the side simply by twisting the body and moving the sword down and to the side.

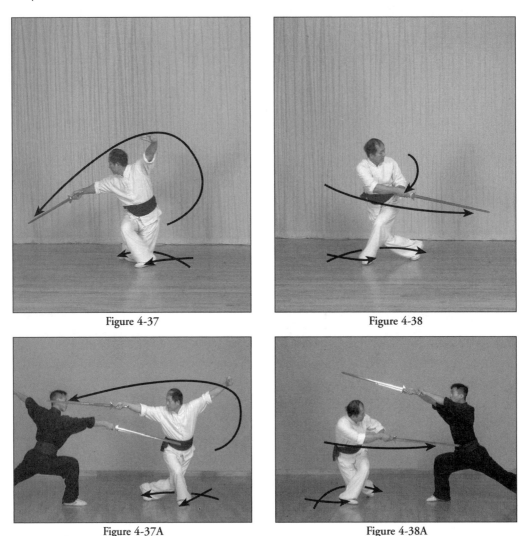

Figure 4-37

Figure 4-38

Figure 4-37A

Figure 4-38A

Figure 4-37: Continue the same motion to the southeast by stepping forward with the right leg and then with the left leg behind the right, still facing southeast, into the crossed leg stance. At the same time move both hands to the chest and chop down with the sword.

Figure 4-37A: After blocking in Figure 4-36A, White takes two steps into the crossed leg stance and attacks Black.

Figure 4-38: Step with the left leg to the northwest while bringing both hands together at the chest. Continue this motion by moving the right foot behind the left to the west and repeat the form shown in Figure 4-9. The sword now points west.

Figure 4-38A: After blocking Black's sword, White steps toward Black and attacks the now open midsection (same as Figure 4-9A).

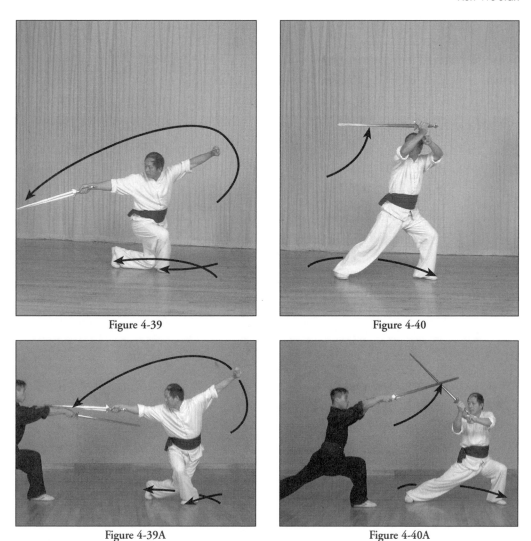

Figure 4-39

Figure 4-40

Figure 4-39A

Figure 4-40A

Figure 4-39: Step to the right with the right leg (east) while bringing both hands together at the chest. Continue this motion to the east as you step with the left leg behind the right into the crossed leg stance. As this step occurs, move the sword in a circular and vertical direction over the head from west to east to the position shown. This is the same ending position as in Figure 4-37.

Figure 4-39A: White steps around Black and chops down at his wrist.

Figure 4-40: Move the left leg to the west into the bow and arrow stance as the left hand joins the right in the position shown.

Figure 4-40A: White guides Black's sword away.

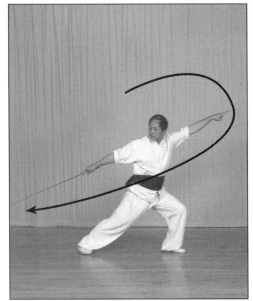

Figure 4-41

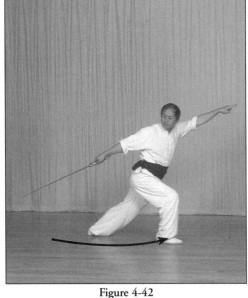

Figure 4-42

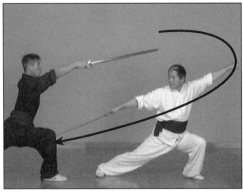

Figure 4-41A

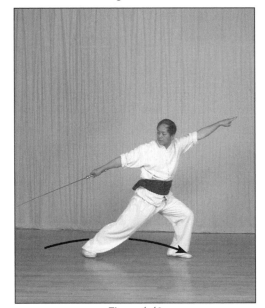

Figure 4-41: In the same stance, move the sword down at a 45 degree angle in a circular motion to point east. The left hand stretches upward and to the west, while looking east.

Figure 4-43

Figure 4-41A: After blocking in Figure 4-40A, White continues the motion and cuts Black's knee.

Figures 4-42 to 4-45: With the arms in the same position take four steps to the west while looking east, ending with the left leg forward in the bow and arrow stance as in Figure 4-41.

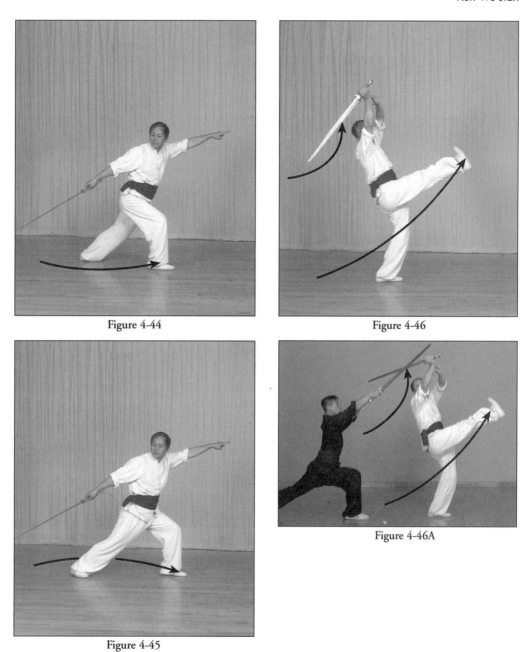

Figure 4-44

Figure 4-46

Figure 4-46A

Figure 4-45

Figure 4-46: Bring the left two fingers to the right wrist and raise the sword, raising the right leg and stretching forward.

Figure 4-46A: White blocks Black's attack from the rear.

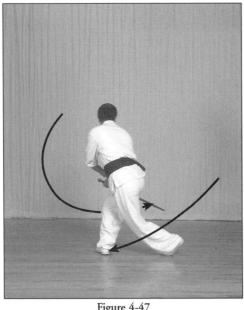

Figure 4-47

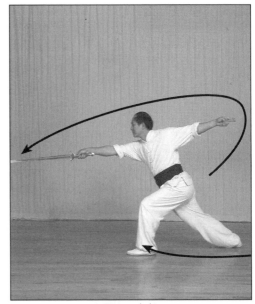
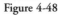

Figure 4-48

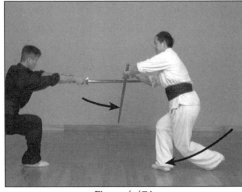

Figure 4-47A

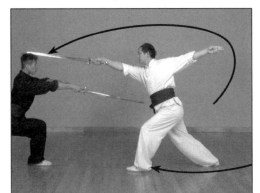

Figure 4-48A

Figure 4-47: Bring the right leg down behind the left and turn the body 180 degrees to the right into the crossed leg stance. The arm positions remain approximately the same as in Figure 4-46, the arms merely drop to the position shown. The body faces east while the sword points west.

Figure 4-47A: White guides Black's sword to the side by turning his body.

Figure 4-48: Continue this motion to the east by stepping forward with the left leg into the bow and arrow stance. As you step forward with the left leg, continue the circular motion of the block by turning the wrist and moving the sword in a vertical circle from west to east to the position shown. The left arm points west.

Figure 4-48A: After blocking in Figure 4-47A, White steps in and chops down at Black's head.

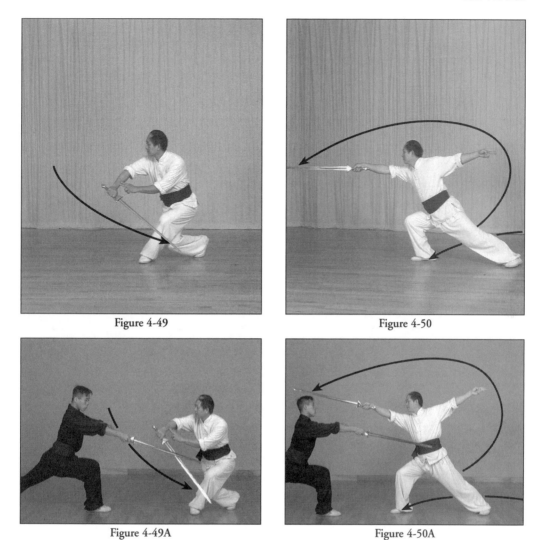

Figure 4-49

Figure 4-50

Figure 4-49A

Figure 4-50A

Figure 4-49: Turn left, shifting into the crossed leg stance with the left foot forward. At the same time lower the sword blade down and to the side while returning the left fingers to the right wrist.

Figure 4-49A: White guides Black's sword away by twisting into the crossed leg stance.

Figure 4-50: Step forward with the right leg into the bow and arrow stance as the sword cuts the enemy with the same motion described in Figure 4-48, except this time the right leg is forward. Again the left hand points west.

Figure 4-50A: After blocking in Figure 4-49A, White steps in and chops down at Black's shoulder.

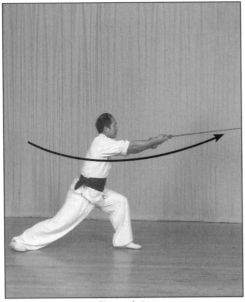

Figure 4-51

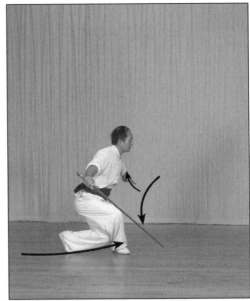

Figure 4-52

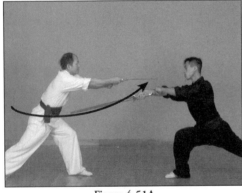

Figure 4-51A

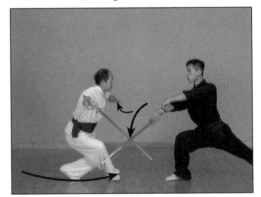

Figure 4-52A

Figure 4-51: Turn left 180 degrees into the bow and arrow stance with the left leg forward while swinging the sword in a horizontal circle with the body to meet the left hand. Again the fingers of the left hand rest on the right wrist.

Figure 4-51A: White cuts Black's neck with his arms outstretched while avoiding Black's attack.

Figure 4-52: Step forward with the right leg into the unicorn stance as the sword swings down and to the side as in Figure 4-32.

Figure 4-52A: White guides Black's attack to the side.

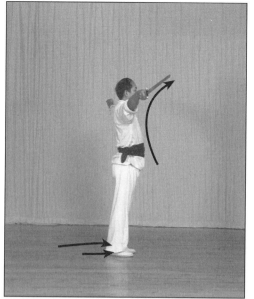

Figure 4-53

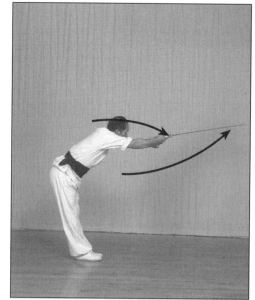

Figure 4-54

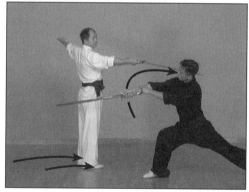

Figure 4-53A

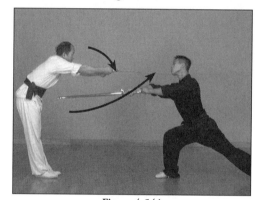

Figure 4-54A

Figure 4-53: Step forward with the left leg as the two hands come together at the stomach. Bring the right leg up beside the left and stand upright. At the same time, raise both hands up in front of the chest, left fingers on right wrist, right palm up, and spread the arms apart now in a horizontal motion ending in the position shown.

Figure 4-53A: After blocking in Figure 4-52A, White steps to the side and cuts Black's neck.

Figure 4-54: Bring both hands together in front of the chest with both arms extended as the stomach withdraws and the chest lowers.

Figure 4-54A: White avoids Black's thrust to the midsection by withdrawing the stomach and at the same time cuts Black's neck.

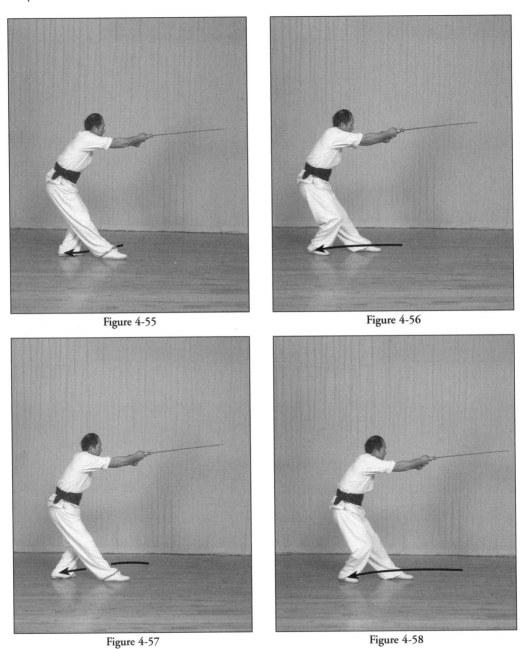

Figure 4-55

Figure 4-56

Figure 4-57

Figure 4-58

Figures 4-55 to 4-59: Keeping the arms in the same position, step back with the left leg first into the false stance. Take five steps backward, ending up with the right leg forward on the fifth step.

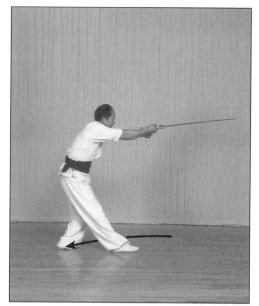

Figure 4-59

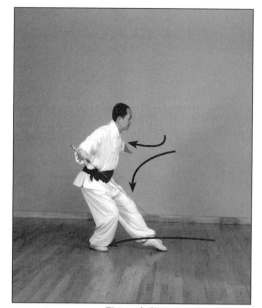

Figure 4-60

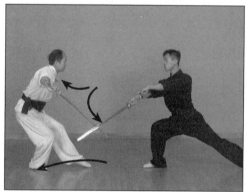

Figure 4-60A

Figure 4-60: Step back with the right leg into the false stance continuing the same motion and move the sword down and to the side, palms facing down.

Figure 4-60A: White finally stops his backward motion and blocks Black's forward thrust.

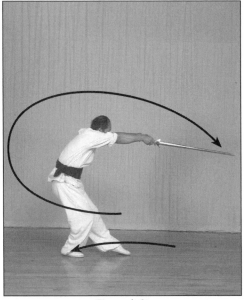

Figure 4-61

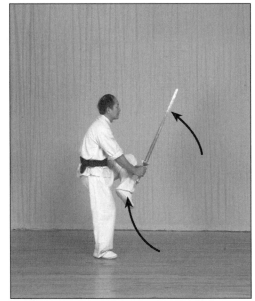

Figure 4-62

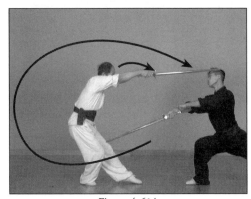

Figure 4-61A

Figure 4-61: Continue the same motion with the sword and raise the arms up beside the body with the arms still outstretched. The left hand points south, while the sword points north. Continue the same motion by raising both arms above the head, where the left fingers touch the right wrist, then bring both arms forward in front of the body with the shoulders raised, extending the sword forward as much as possible.

Figure 4-61A: White cuts Black's head while stretching to avoid Black's attack.

Figure 4-62: Move the sword in toward the body as the left leg rises into the golden rooster stands on one leg stance, while touching the left fingers to the right wrist.

Figure 4-63: Step forward with the left leg and thrust the sword forward.

Figure 4-64: Move the sword back to the body as in Figure 4-62, but remain in the bow and arrow stance.

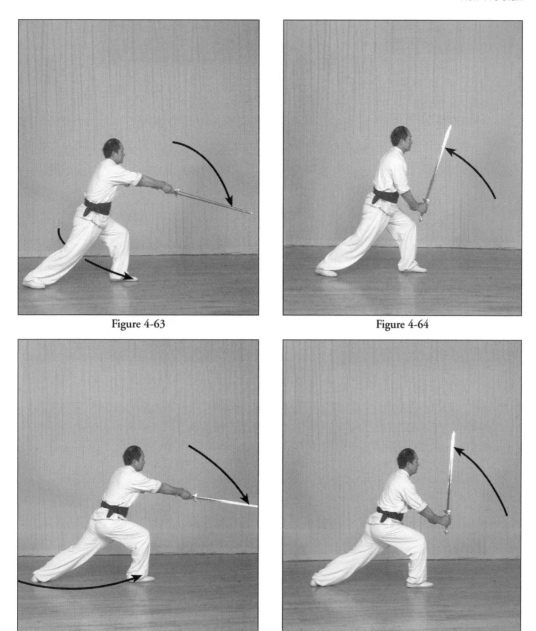

Figure 4-63

Figure 4-64

Figure 4-65

Figure 4-66

Figure 4-65: Step forward with the right leg into the bow and arrow stance and thrust the sword forward.

Figures 4-66 to 4-69: Continue stepping, blocking, and thrusting two more times. Including Figures 4-62 to 4-65, there should be four steps, blocks, and thrusts, ending with the right leg forward in the bow and arrow stance as shown in Figure 4-69.

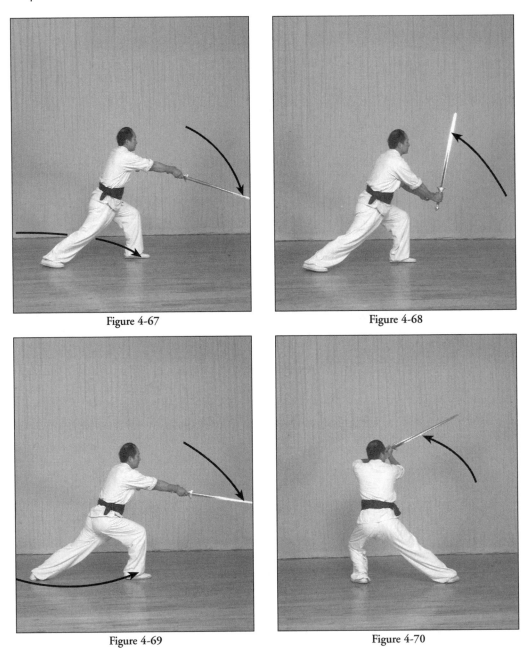

Figure 4-67

Figure 4-68

Figure 4-69

Figure 4-70

Figure 4-70: Shift the weight to the left leg into the taming the tiger stance. Raise the sword to the southeast as shown. This form is the same as Figure 4-27.

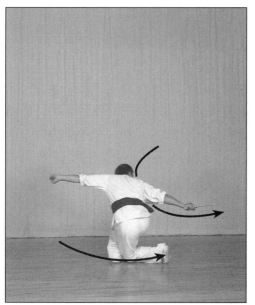

Figure 4-71

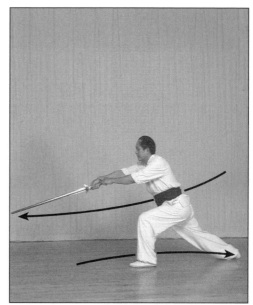

Figure 4-72

Figure 4-71: Move the left foot behind and to the west of the right foot into the crossed leg stance. At the same time, point east with the left hand while cutting down and forward at a 45 degree angle with the sword, palm down. This form is the same as Figure 4-28.

Figure 4-72: Move the right leg backward into the bow and arrow stance facing east with the left leg forward. At the same time return the left fingers to the right wrist and thrust the sword forward, slightly downward to the east.

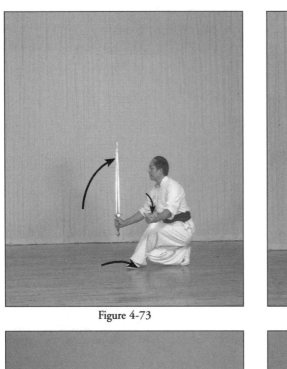

Figure 4-73

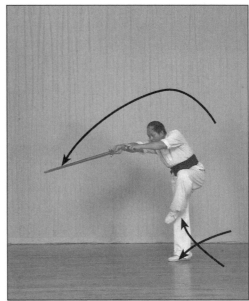

Figure 4-74

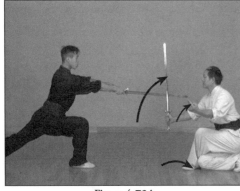

Figure 4-73A

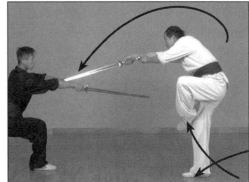

Figure 4-74A

Figure 4-73: Sit down into the crossed leg stance facing east as the sword handle moves down and the sword tip comes back toward the body. The left hand moves down and to the side, palm up.

Figure 4-73A: White guides Black's sword to the side as the sword handle is lowered.

Figure 4-74: Stand up with the weight on the left leg and raise the right leg slightly. Then hop toward southeast onto the right leg while raising the left knee. At the same time bring both hands together at the chest and thrust the sword forward while the hop onto the right leg is made. The upper body leans forward for added extension of the sword.

Figure 4-74A: White hops up in order to attack Black's arms from above.

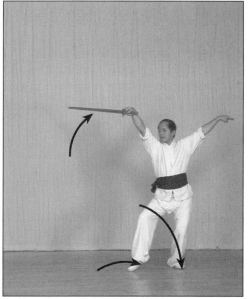

Figure 4-75

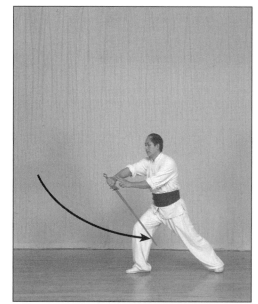

Figure 4-76

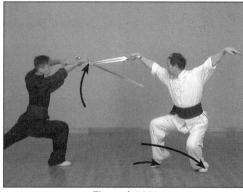

Figure 4-75A

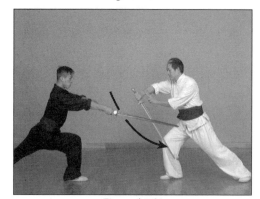

Figure 4-76A

Figure 4-75: Hop back with the left leg to the west into the false stance with the right leg forward and pointing east. While hopping back, the sword rises very slightly to the position shown and the left hand points back to the west.

Figure 4-75A: White cuts Black's wrists from below.

Figure 4-76: Step forward with the right leg and move the sword down and to the left side of the body as you touch the right wrist with the left fingers.

Figure 4-76A: White guides Black's sword to the side while moving forward and twisting the body slightly to the left.

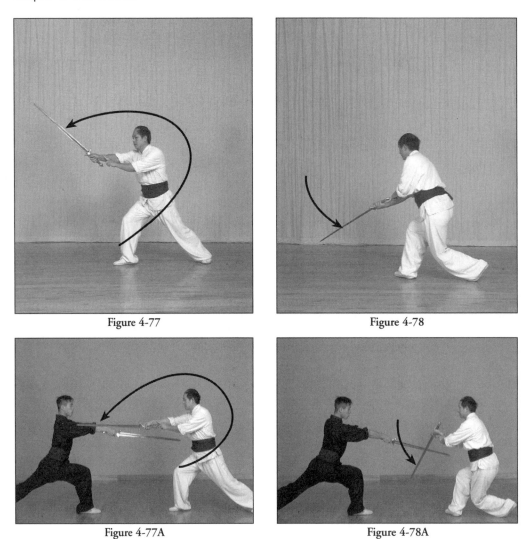

Figure 4-77

Figure 4-78

Figure 4-77A

Figure 4-78A

Figure 4-77: Continue the sword motion clockwise, cutting down to the east.

Figure 4-77A: White continues the sword motion from Figure 4-76A and cuts Black's wrist.

Figure 4-78: Shift into the crossed leg stance and bring the sword down and to the right as the body twists to the right. End with the right palm facing away from the body.

Figure 4-78A: By twisting his body, White blocks Black's weapon by guiding the forward force to the side.

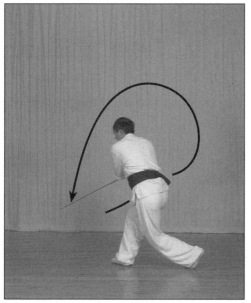

Figure 4-79

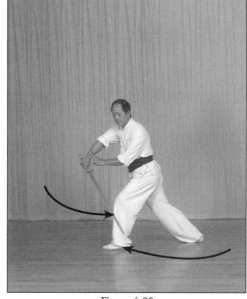

Figure 4-80

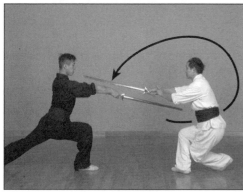

Figure 4-79A

Figure 4-79: Continue the sword motion counterclockwise, cutting down to the southeast.

Figure 4-79A: White continues the sword motion from Figure 4-78A and cuts Black's wrist.

Figure 4-80: Step forward with the left leg while turning the wrist counterclockwise, so that the right palm faces down. The chest faces south.

179

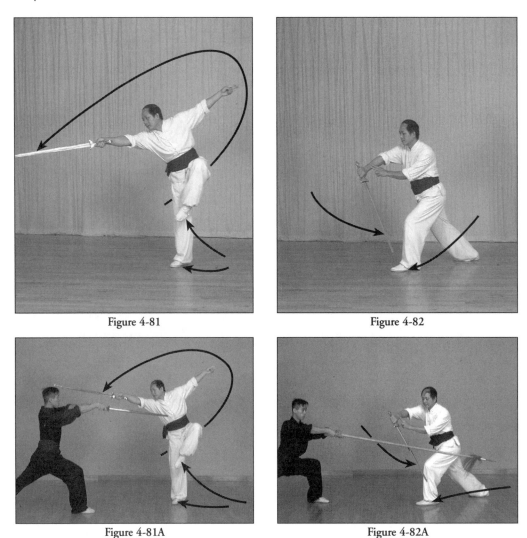

Figure 4-81

Figure 4-82

Figure 4-81A

Figure 4-82A

Figure 4-81: Continue this same motion by raising the right leg, and then spring off with the left leg and turn the body 180 degrees in the air. Land with the left leg up. During the jump, the sword moves in a large circle from the position in Figure 4-80 at a 45 degree angle up and then down to the position shown. During this cut, the left arm points up and to the west.

Figure 4-81A: After blocking, White jumps and spins to the right, and cuts Black.

Figure 4-82: Step left leg forward into the bow and arrow stance and at the same time move the sword down.

Figure 4-82A: White guides Black's spear attack to the side and downward.

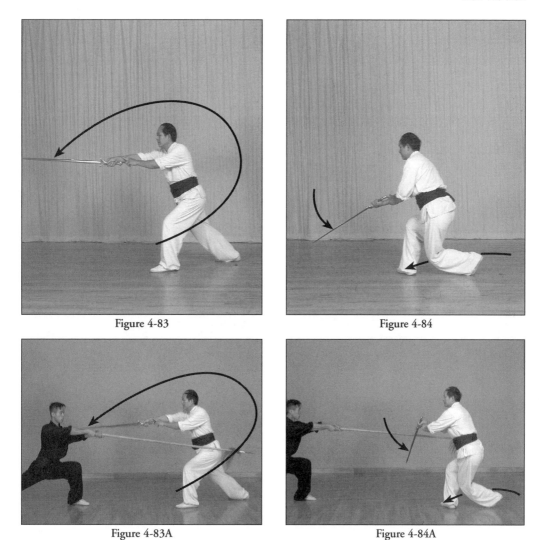

Figure 4-83

Figure 4-84

Figure 4-83A

Figure 4-84A

Figure 4-83: Continue the sword motion clockwise and cut down vertically.

Figure 4-83A: After blocking in Figure 4-82A, White cuts Black's wrist.

Figure 4-84: Step right leg forward into the crossed leg stance and bring the sword down and to the right as the body twists to the right.

Figure 4-84A: White blocks Black's weapon by guiding the spear to the side.

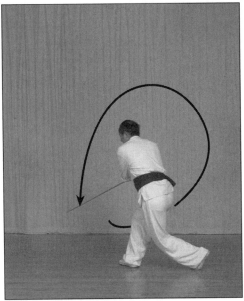

Figure 4-85

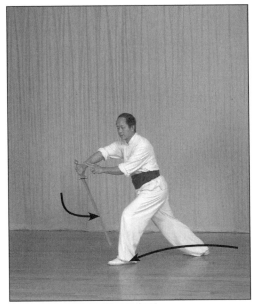

Figure 4-86

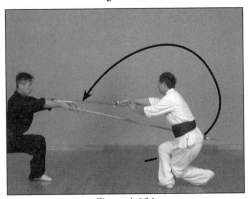

Figure 4-85A

Figure 4-85: Continue the sword motion clockwise and cut down to the southwest.

Figure 4-85A: White continues the sword motion from Figure 4-84A and cuts Black's wrist.

Figure 4-86: The same as Figure 4-80.

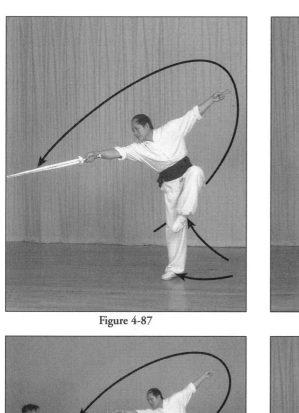

Figure 4-87

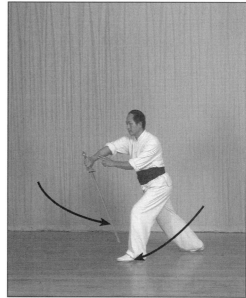

Figure 4-88

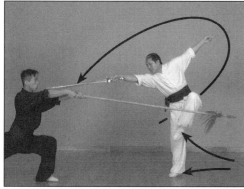

Figure 4-87A

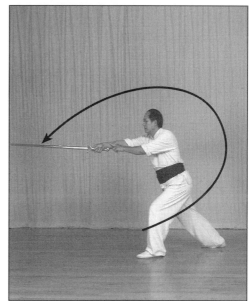

Figure 4-89

Figure 4-87: The same as Figure 4-81.

Figure 4-87A: White chops down to Black's shoulder.

Figures 4-88 to 4-93: Repeat the motions from Figures 4-82 to 4-87. In all, there are three jumps and spins.

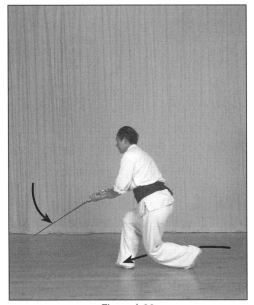

Figure 4-90

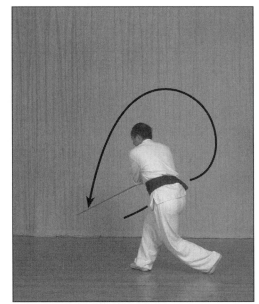

Figure 4-91

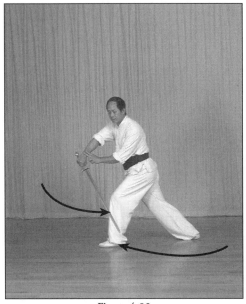

Figure 4-92

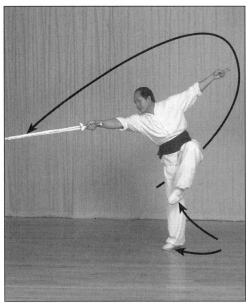

Figure 4-93

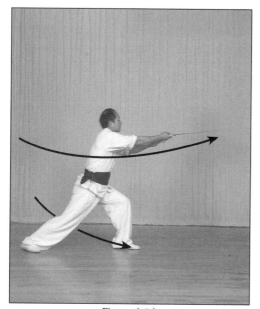

Figure 4-94

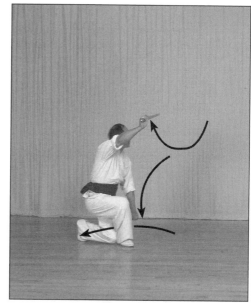

Figure 4-95

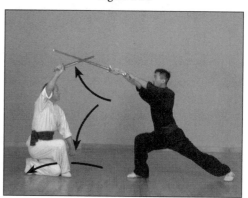

Figure 4-95A

Figure 4-94: Step back to the west with the left leg and turn left into the bow and arrow stance, while swinging the sword and the left arm in a horizontal motion with the right palm up to the position shown.

Figure 4-95: Step back into the unicorn stance with the left leg. At the same time turn the point of the sword to the left and lower the left hand. The right palm faces forward.

Figure 4-95A: White avoids Black's attack by sitting low and protecting himself by turning his sword to the position shown and guiding Black's sword above his head.

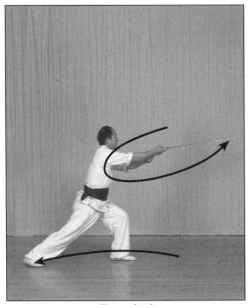

Figure 4-96

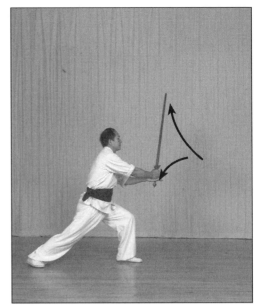

Figure 4-97

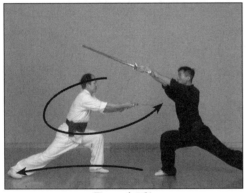

Figure 4-96A

Figure 4-96: Step back with the right leg into the bow and arrow stance while swinging the sword horizontally to the left into the position shown. The right wrist faces up with the left fingers touching it.

Figure 4-96A: After blocking in Figure 4-95A, White steps back and cuts Black's midsection.

Figure 4-97: Swing the sword down and to the left, then turn the wrist clockwise. At the same time, the left hand grasps the sword hilt.

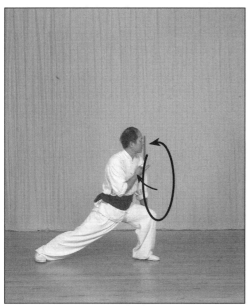

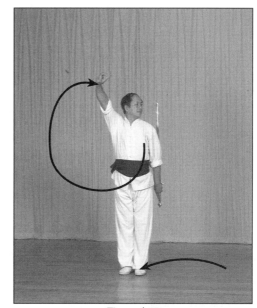

Figure 4-98   Figure 4-99

Figure 4-98: Take the sword with the left hand, fingers pointing toward the butt of the sword. Lower the left hand, turning the wrist clockwise, and end with the fingers pointing to the ground, palm facing to the rear, and sword pointing straight up. At the same time bring the right hand to the stomach, palm up in the secret sword position.

Figure 4-99: Bring the left leg back beside the right while turning 90 degrees to the right; stand upright facing north. At the same time circle the right hand counterclockwise to the right to point down, by the side, then continue the circle and hold the hand overhead. Look to the left.

CHAPTER 5

Qi Men Jian

戚門劍

5-1. INTRODUCTION

One of the most famous of the long sword sequences is the Qi family's sword sequence, which employs a number of advanced techniques coordinated with leg movements. Learning this sequence is a long, painful process, and the two sequences already presented must be learned first.

The sequence was created by Qi, Ji-Guang (戚繼光), who was born in 1528 A.D. during the Ming Dynasty (明朝) at Dong Mou Xian in Shandong Province (山東、東牟縣). He studied the martial arts from early childhood on. His father, Qi, Jing-Tong (戚景東), was an official in Deng Zhou (登州) in charge of guarding the city. Qi, Jing-Tong was a man of great integrity, loyal to his parents and emperor. In short, an honest official. Once his father asked Qi, Ji-Guang what he wanted to be when he grew up, and he replied that he wanted to be clean living, honest, loyal, and filial. When he was ten, his mother died. Then, when he was 17, his father died also, and Qi, Ji-Guang assumed his father's position.

From the time of the Han Dynasty in 2 A.D. (漢朝) until the Yuan Dynasty (1206-1368 A.D., 元朝), pirates from Japan had paid tribute to the Chinese emperor in order to be able to carry out raids, unmolested by the Chinese military. The emperor Kublai Khan of the Yuan Dynasty invaded Japan when his emissaries were executed by the Japanese Shogun, but the invasion failed. From that time the pirates stopped paying tribute to the emperor, and continued raiding the Chinese coast, much like the Vikings in medieval Europe. These raids continued until the beginning of the Ming Dynasty.

In 1555 A.D. at the age of 27, Qi, Ji-Guang was assigned to put a stop to these raids. He pursued this task over a long period of time and completed it before he died at the age of 61 in 1589. In order to do this he trained and maintained an army, and had the reputation of being very strict in his training. Besides the sword sequence presented here, he is known for having written two books, the *Book of Efficient Discipline* (*Ji Xiao Xin Shu,* 紀效新書) and the *Record of Practical Training of Soldiers*

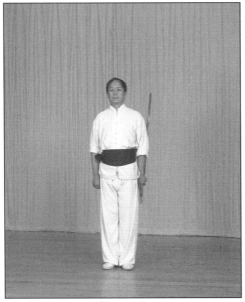

Figure 5-1

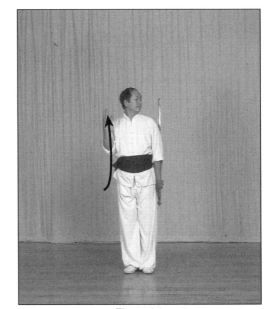

Figure 5-2

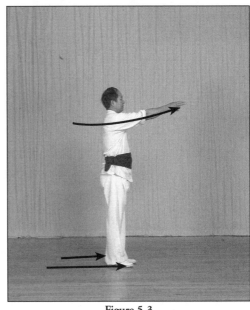

Figure 5-3

(*Lian Bing Shi Ji,* 練兵實紀). These books contain the fighting strategies and a number of the martial techniques in use at that time.

In the next section, the Qi sword sequence will be illustrated with the person in the white shirt demonstrating the solo form, while the person in the black shirt acts as the attacker in the applications of the forms. The first level solution of every technique will be given. In the description of the moves, the direction originally faced is considered North.

5-2 QI MEN JIAN

Figure 5-1: Stand upright facing north holding the sword with the left hand, palms facing south.

Figure 5-2: Raise the right hand up to the position shown in the secret sword form with the extended fingers pointing up. Look left to the west as the arm is raised.

Figure 5-3: Turn the body 90 degrees left to face west while stepping to the west with the left foot. Move the right foot up next to the left and extend the right hand to a horizontal position to point west in front of the body.

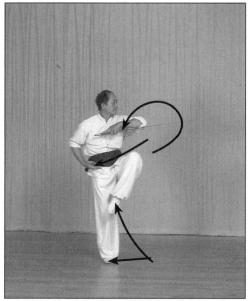

Figure 5-4

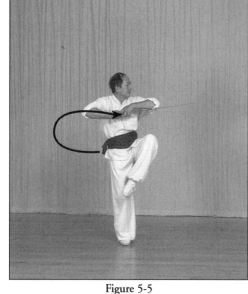

Figure 5-5

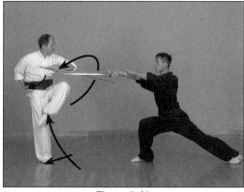

Figure 5-4A

Figure 5-4: Step back with the right leg and raise the left leg to the position shown. As the right leg moves back, drop the right hand to the waist, palm up. As the left leg rises, raise the left arm straight out to point west and then swing the arm in toward the chest so that the sword points west. The left palm faces down.

Figure 5-4A: White steps back and blocks Black's attack by moving the sword from left to right.

Figure 5-5: Swing the right arm straight out to point east and, continuing this motion, bring it back to the chest and grasp the underside of the sword handle.

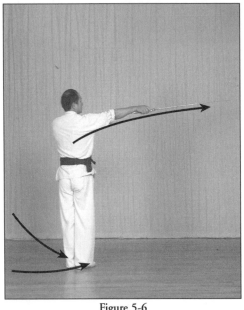

Figure 5-6

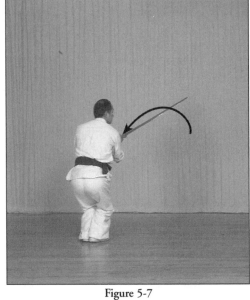

Figure 5-7

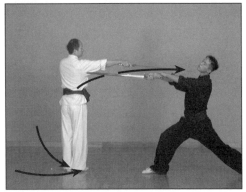

Figure 5-6A

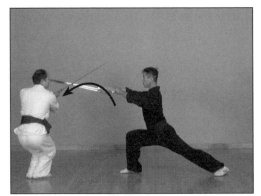

Figure 5-7A

Figure 5-6: Take two steps forward, first with the left leg, then with the right as shown. As you step forward with the right leg, turn the body 90 degrees to the left to face south. At the same time thrust the sword forward to the right side, right palm down. The left hand concurrently moves in front of the right armpit in the secret sword position, palm down.

Figure 5-6A: After blocking Black's thrust, White steps in toward Black to the side of his sword and attacks.

Figure 5-7: Bring the right hand back to the chest with the palm facing the body, bend the knees, and lower the body. Left fingers touch the right wrist.

Figure 5-7A: White's sword follows Black's sword in as Black attacks, and guides it to the side.

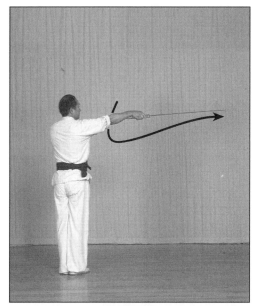

Figure 5-8

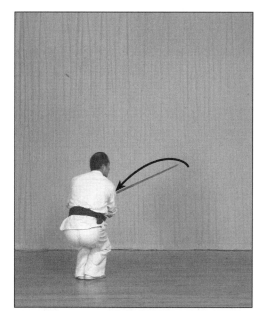

Figure 5-9

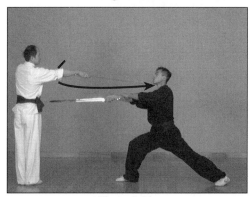

Figure 5-8A

Figure 5-8: Stand upright again and thrust the sword to the right once again, right palm down.

Figure 5-8A: After blocking in Figure 5-7A, White slides in to attack Black.

Figures 5-9 to 5-12: Repeat Figures 5-7 and 5-8 twice.

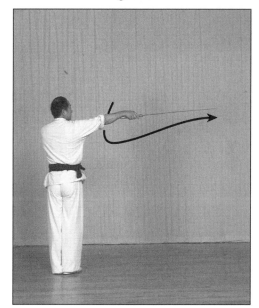

Figure 5-10

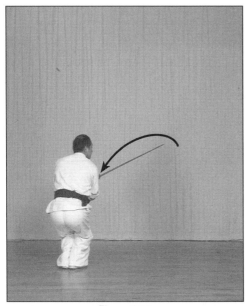

Figure 5-11

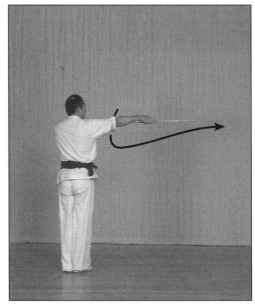

Figure 5-12

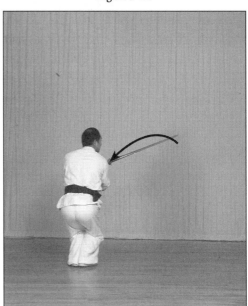

Figure 5-13

Figure 5-13: Repeat Figure 5-7.

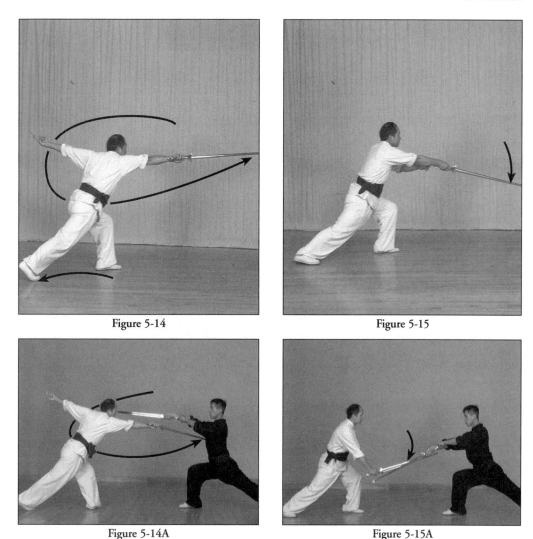

Figure 5-14

Figure 5-15

Figure 5-14A

Figure 5-15A

Figure 5-14: Stretch the right leg back behind the left with only the toes touching the ground. At the same time continue this motion by rotating the sword in a vertical circle so that the tip moves up, to the rear, down, and then forward again with the left hand stretching to the rear (east) and both palms facing north.

Figure 5-14A: After blocking in Figure 5-13. White attacks Black's arms by striking from underneath.

Figure 5-15: Step down on the right heel and change the stance to the bow and arrow stance. At the same time bring the fingers of the left hand to the right wrist and lower the sword slightly.

Figure 5-15A: Moving the sword down blocks the enemy's attack.

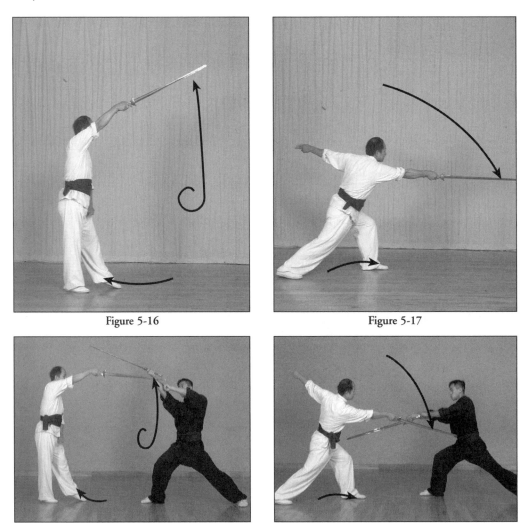

Figure 5-16

Figure 5-17

Figure 5-16A

Figure 5-17A

Figure 5-16: Rotate the right hand counterclockwise in a small circle quickly, and raise the sword as you shift all the weight to the right leg and withdraw the left to touch with the toes only. The left hand moves to the abdomen, palm facing in.

Figure 5-16A: As White presses his sword down in Figure 5-15A, he circles the sword and slices up at Black's wrist.

Figure 5-17: Step forward (west) with the left leg into the bow and arrow stance again as the sword chops down to the position shown. At the same time point to the rear with the left hand.

Figure 5-17A: White chops down at Black's wrist or body.

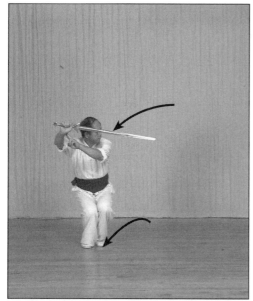

Figure 5-18

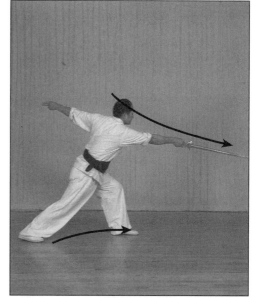

Figure 5-19

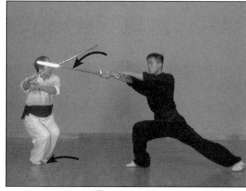

Figure 5-18A

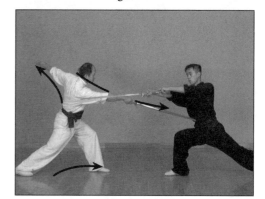

Figure 5-19A

Figure 5-18: Move the left foot back next to the right into a very low stance as you rotate the body 90 degrees to the right. All the weight is on the right foot. Bring the left hand to the right wrist as the right arm follows the body back. As the right arm withdraws, rotate the wrist counterclockwise so that the right palm ends up facing north, as does the body. This is all one smooth motion. Look to the west as the body faces north.

Figure 5-18A: As Black thrusts his sword toward him, White withdraws his body and guides Black's sword to the side.

Figure 5-19: Step to the west again with the left leg into the bow and arrow stance, and thrust the sword forward, pointing to the rear with the left hand.

Figure 5-19A: After blocking in Figure 5-18A, White slides his sword along Black's sword and steps in to stab Black's waist.

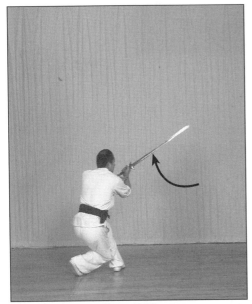

Figure 5-20

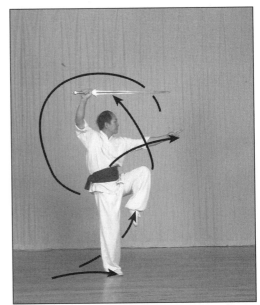

Figure 5-21

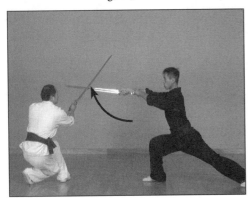

Figure 5-20A

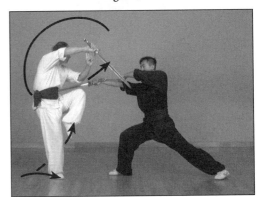

Figure 5-21A

Figure 5-20: Rotate the right wrist clockwise as you rotate the upper body to the left into the crossed leg stance and withdraw the sword to the left. At the same time move the left hand to the right wrist.

Figure 5-20A: White guides Black's attack away and to the side.

Figure 5-21: Lower the right hand and rotate the right wrist so that the sword tip travels in a vertical circle, first traveling up, to the rear, down, forward, and then up again to the position shown. While making the circle with the sword, step forward with the right leg, and then raise the left leg up to the position shown just as the body twists and the sword moves to the position shown. The left hand points forward as the leg is raised. You are facing west at this point.

Figure 5-21A: After blocking in Figure 5-20A, White steps toward Black and slices Black's chest.

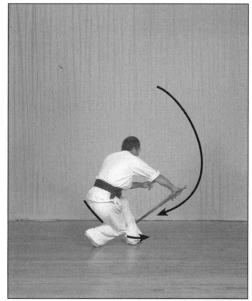

Figure 5-22

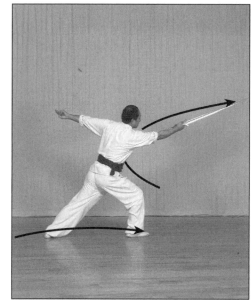

Figure 5-23

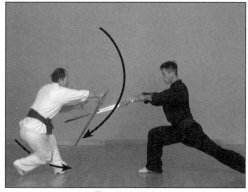

Figure 5-22A

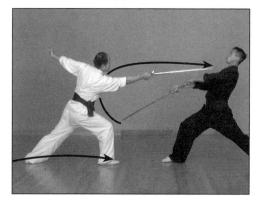

Figure 5-23A

Figure 5-22: Step down with the left leg and twist the body to the left into the crossed leg stance as the sword tip travels forward, down, and then to the rear in a circular motion into the position shown. The left hand moves to the right wrist.

Figure 5-22A: White guides Black's attack away with the motions described above.

Figure 5-23: Continue the circular motion of the sword backward, upward, and then forward. Step forward with the right leg into the bow and arrow stance.

Figure 5-23A: White would counter the attack by continuing to circle the sword up from the position shown in Figure 5-22A and then forward to the head or throat.

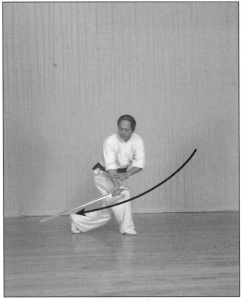

Figure 5-24

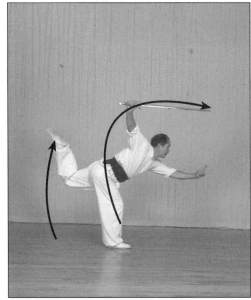

Figure 5-25

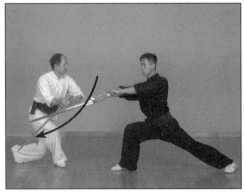

Figure 5-24A

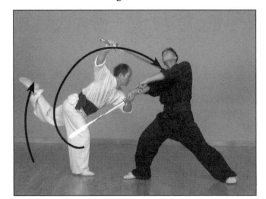

Figure 5-25A

Figure 5-24: Twist the body to the right into the crossed leg stance as you lower the sword tip down and to the right and then to the rear.

Figure 5-24A: White guides Black's attack away with the motions described above.

Figure 5-25: Continue the same circular motion with the sword tip as the tip travels up over the head and then forward as you raise the left leg and lean forward. Point the left hand forward.

Figure 5-25A: After blocking in Figure 5-24A, White slides by Black's sword and stabs Black's throat.

Figure 5-26: Step forward with the left leg into the bow and arrow stance and thrust the sword forward (west). The left hand points to the rear.

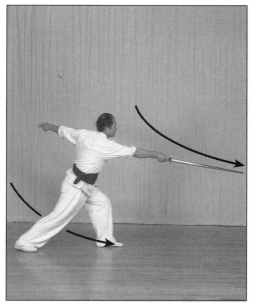

Figure 5-26

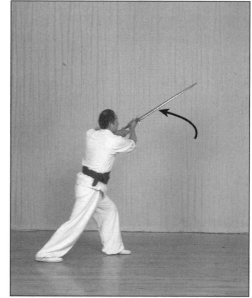

Figure 5-27

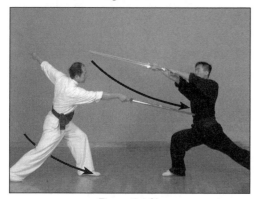

Figure 5-26A

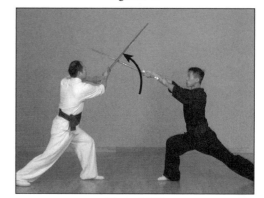

Figure 5-27A

Figure 5-26A: White ducks under Black's attack by stepping low into the bow and arrow stance and attacks Black's midsection.

Figure 5-27: Rotate the right wrist clockwise as you rotate the upper body and withdraw the sword to the left. At the same time move the left hand to the right wrist.

Figure 5-27A: White guides Black's attack away and to the side.

Figure 5-28: Step forward (west) with the right leg and then step west with the left leg behind the right into the crossed leg stance as the sword moves in a chop to the position shown. The body is facing south and the left hand points in the opposite direction from the sword.

Figure 5-28A: After blocking in Figure 5-27A, White steps in toward Black and chops down at a 45 degree angle to Black's leg as shown.

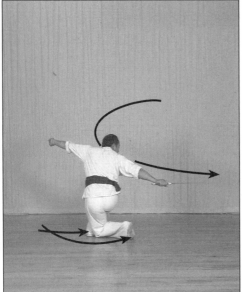

Figure 5-28

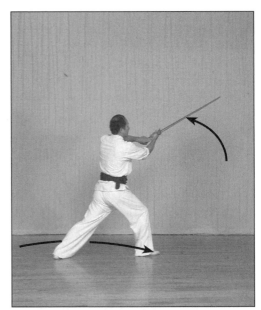

Figure 5-29

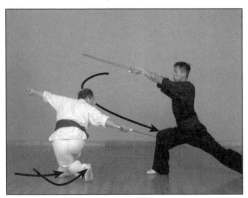

Figure 5-28A

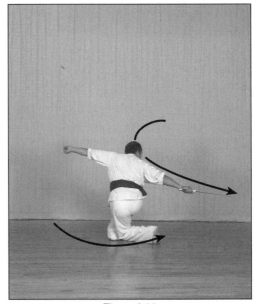

Figure 5-30

Figures 5-29 and 5-30: Repeat Figures 5-27 and 5-28.

Figure 5-31: Step to the west with the right leg into the bow and arrow stance as you raise the sword over the head and then chop down with the sword to the position shown. The left hand moves to the right wrist.

Figure 5-31A: White chops down at Black's wrists as Black attempts to attack. Or, White pushes down Black's sword to stop Black's attack.

Figure 5-32: Rotate the right hand counterclockwise in a small circle quickly, and raise the sword as you shift your weight to the right leg and withdraw the left so that only the toes are touching. The left hand moves to the abdomen, palm down and pointing south.

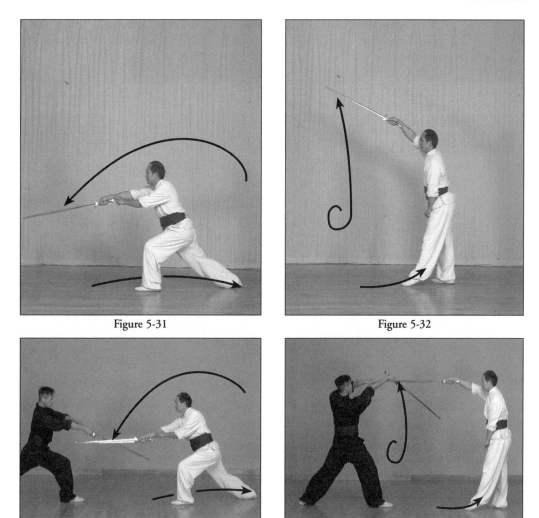

Figure 5-31

Figure 5-32

Figure 5-31A

Figure 5-32A

Figure 5-32A: As White raises his sword, he slices up at Black's wrist. The counterclockwise rotation of the right hand slides Black's sword slightly to the south to make the opening for slicing the wrist.

Figure 5-33: Step forward (east) with the left leg into the bow and arrow stance again as the sword chops down to the position shown. At the same time point to the rear with the left hand.

Figure 5-33A: White chops down at Black's body.

Figure 5-34: Keeping the same stance, rotate the right wrist clockwise and drop the tip of the sword down and to the right. The right palm faces up and the left hand moves to the right wrist.

Figure 5-34A: With this motion White directs Black's chop down to the right.

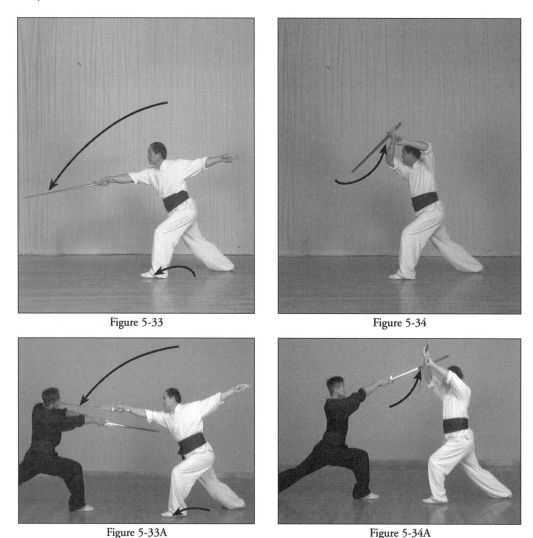

Figure 5-33

Figure 5-34

Figure 5-33A

Figure 5-34A

Figure 5-35: Step forward (east) with the right leg and rotate the right wrist so that the sword tip travels in a vertical circle up, forward, down and then slightly to the rear. The left foot touches at the toes only. The right palm faces north.

Figures 5-35A and 5-35B: White guides Black's weapon to his right.

Figure 5-36: Step forward with the left leg into the bow and arrow stance and chop down with the sword.

Figures 5-36A and 5-36B: White chops down at Black after blocking in Figures 5-35A and 5-35B.

Figure 5-37: Repeat Figure 5-34.

Figure 5-38: Raise the right leg and then jump up by springing off with the left leg as the sword travels in a circular motion as in Figure 5-35. This form is the same as in Figure 5-35, except you circle the sword while you are in the air.

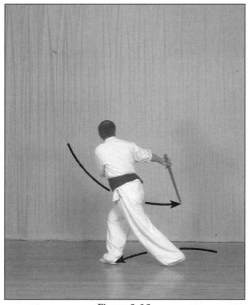

Figure 5-35

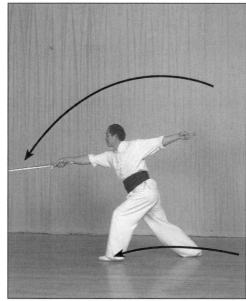

Figure 5-36

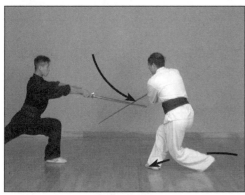

Figure 5-35A

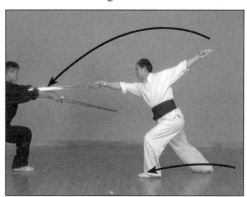

Figure 5-36A

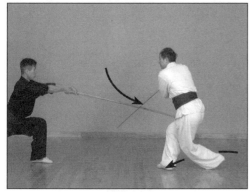

Figure 5-35B

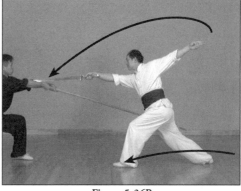

Figure 5-36B

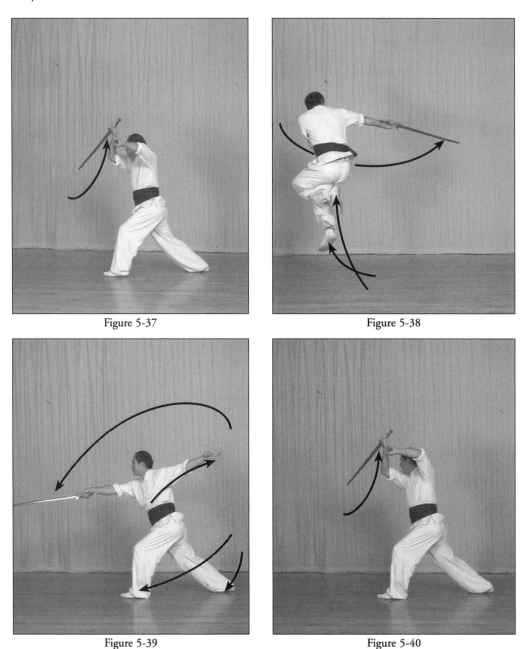

Figure 5-37

Figure 5-38

Figure 5-39

Figure 5-40

Figure 5-39: Repeat Figure 5-33. Land on the right foot and then step forward with the left into the bow and arrow stance as the sword chops down to the position shown. At the same time point to the rear with the left hand.

Figure 5-40: Repeat Figure 5-34.

Figure 5-41: Step forward with the right leg as you rotate your right wrist counterclockwise and move the sword tip in a vertical circle to the rear, up, forward, and

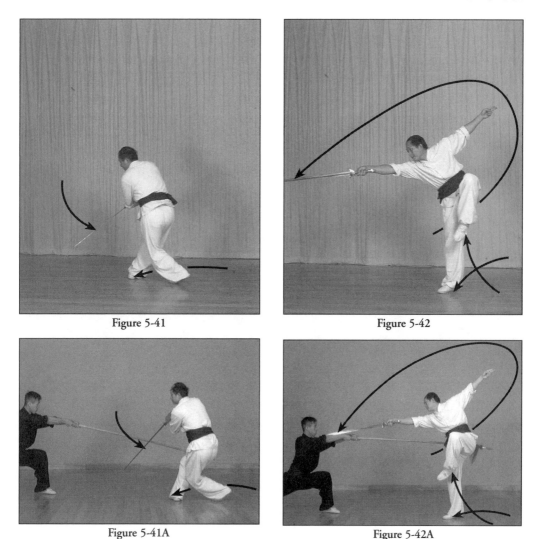

Figure 5-41

Figure 5-42

Figure 5-41A

Figure 5-42A

finally down to the position shown. The right palm faces to the rear; the left hand is held on the right wrist, while the left foot touches at the toes only.

Figure 5-41A: White guides Black's weapon to the side as he steps in toward Black.

Figure 5-42: From Figure 5-41, take two steps forward to the east, first with the left and then with the right leg, at the same time turn the body to the right 180 degrees until the body faces north. As you step down with the right foot, the left foot is raised and the sword travels 180 degrees in a circular motion and chops down. The left hand points in the opposite direction from the sword.

Figure 5-42A: White continues his blocking motion by continuing the same motion with the sword and stepping closer to Black in a circular fashion to finally chop down at Black's shoulder.

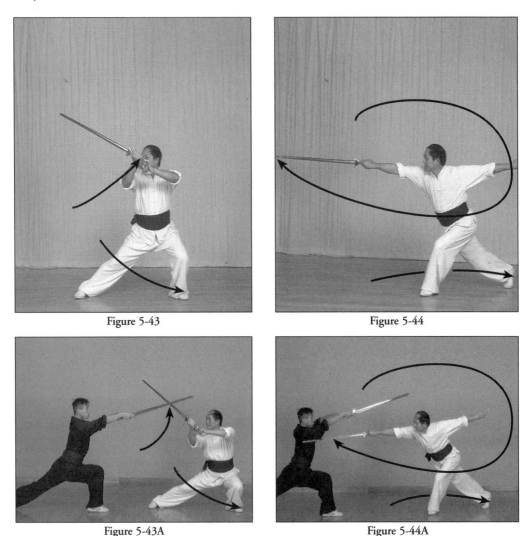

Figure 5-43

Figure 5-44

Figure 5-43A

Figure 5-44A

Figure 5-43: Step down and back to the west with the left leg, and rotate the right wrist clockwise as you withdraw the sword. The right palm faces south, the chest faces north. The left hand returns to the right wrist.

Figure 5-43A: White guides Black's attack to the side by rotating his wrist and withdrawing the sword.

Figure 5-44: Continuing the same motion, step back and stretch the right leg back behind the left with only the toes touching the ground. At the same time continue this motion by rotating the sword in a vertical circle so that the tip moves up, to the rear, down, and then forward again with the left hand stretched to the rear (west) and both palms facing south as shown.

Figure 5-44A: After deflecting Black's attack, White continues the motion and cuts upward.

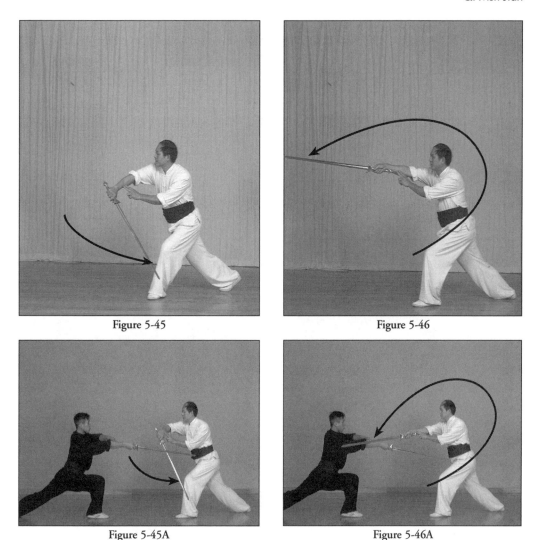

Figure 5-45

Figure 5-46

Figure 5-45A

Figure 5-46A

Figure 5-45: Keeping the same stance, move the tip of the sword down and to the left rear as the left hand returns to the right wrist.

Figure 5-45A: White guides Black's attack away and to the left.

Figure 5-46: Continuing the same circular motion, move the tip of the sword up over the head, and then down to the position shown. The right palm faces north.

Figure 5-46A: After blocking in Figure 5-45A, White continues his motion and chops down at Black's arms.

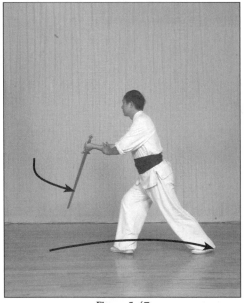

Figure 5-47

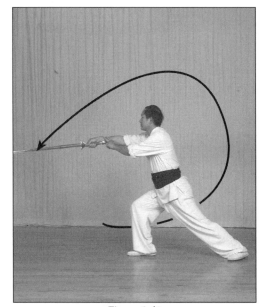

Figure 5-48

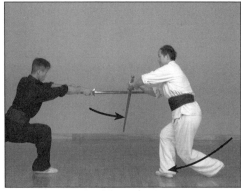

Figure 5-47A

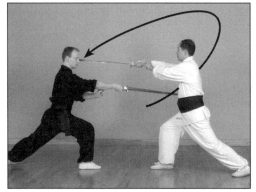

Figure 5-48A

Figure 5-47: Continuing the above motion, step the left leg backward into the bow and arrow stance, twist the body to the right and rotate the right wrist counterclockwise, moving the sword tip down and to the right, with the right palm facing south.

Figure 5-47A: White steps backward with the left leg, and guides Black's attack away and to the right.

Figure 5-48: Continuing the same circular motion, move the tip of the sword up over the head, and then down to the position shown. The right palm faces north.

Figure 5-48A: After blocking, White continues his motion and chops down at Black's shoulder.

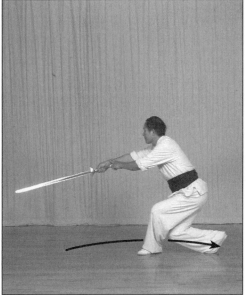

Figure 5-49

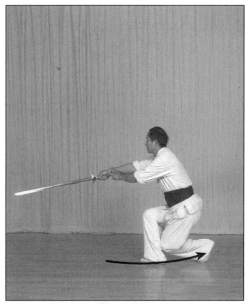

Figure 5-50

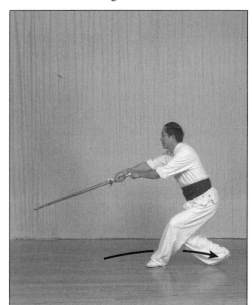

Figure 5-51

Figure 5-49: Keeping the same form,
step back to the west with the right leg into the unicorn stance.

Figure 5-50: Keeping the same form, step back to the west with the left leg into the unicorn stance.

Figure 5-51: Repeat Figure 5-49.

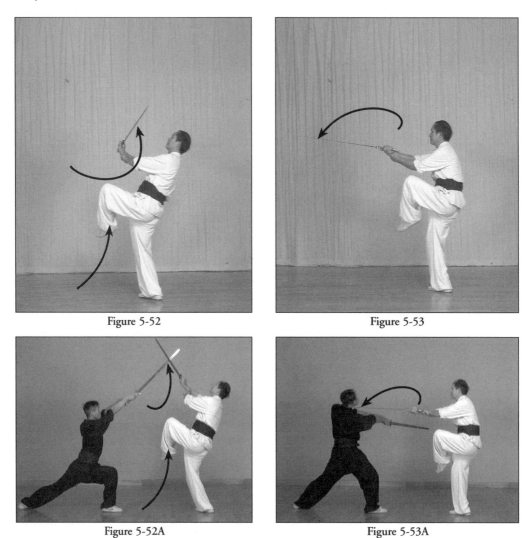

Figure 5-52

Figure 5-53

Figure 5-52A

Figure 5-53A

Figure 5-52: Raise the left leg and lean back. At the same time rotate the right wrist as the sword tip travels down, to the left, and then up and to the right in front of the face. The right palm faces away from the body.

Figure 5-52A: White leans back to avoid Black's attack and blocks Black's sword.

Figure 5-53: Continue this circular motion with the sword so that the tip travels to the right, and then forward to the position shown.

Figure 5-53A: After blocking in Figure 5-52A, White continues his motion and cuts Black's neck.

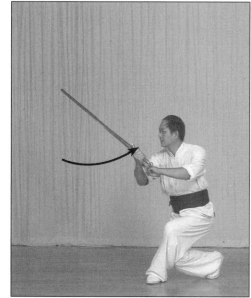
Figure 5-54

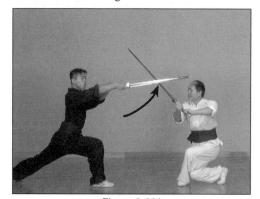
Figure 5-55

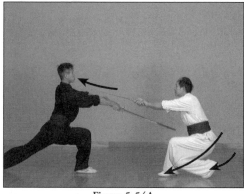
Figure 5-54A

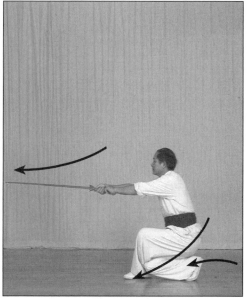
Figure 5-55A

Figure 5-54: Step down with the left foot into the unicorn stance and thrust the sword forward, palm up.

Figure 5-54A: White moves in toward Black and stabs Black's throat.

Figure 5-55: Rotate the right wrist clockwise and withdraw the sword as the body twists to the left. The right palm faces south.

Figure 5-55A: White guides Black's attack away and to the left.

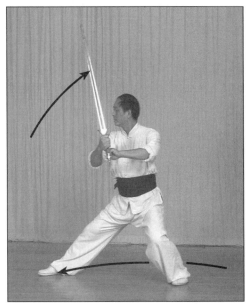

Figure 5-56

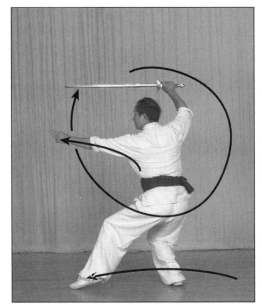

Figure 5-57

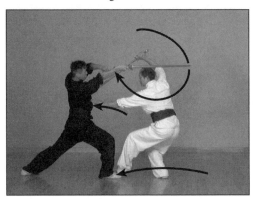

Figure 5-57A

Figure 5-56: Step forward to the east with the right leg and lower the sword hand to the position shown.

Figure 5-57: Continuing the same motion, step forward with the left leg into the false stance and move the sword handle down, forward, and then up to the position shown. The left hand points forward.

Figure 5-57A: White steps in low under Black's attack and slices up at Black's arms.

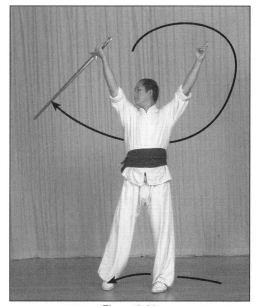

Figure 5-58

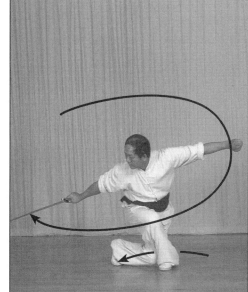

Figure 5-59

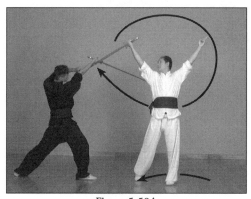

Figure 5-58A

Figure 5-58: Step forward to the east with the right leg and stand upright, with the body facing north and the right foot touching at the toes only. At the same time, move the sword in a circular motion so that the tip travels up, to the rear, and down. The sword tip remains down as the body stands upright, the right wrist faces up.

Figure 5-58A: White steps in and slide cuts Black's arm.

Figure 5-59: Rotate the right wrist counterclockwise as you rotate the upper body to the left and withdraw the sword. At the same time move the left hand to the right wrist. Step forward (east) with the right leg and then step to the east with the left leg behind the right into the crossed leg stance as the sword moves in a chop to the position shown. The body is facing north and the left hand points in the opposite direction from the sword. The right palm faces down.

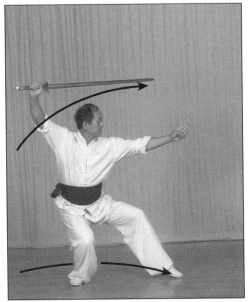

Figure 5-60

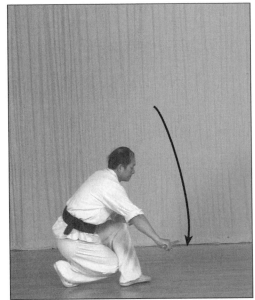

Figure 5-61

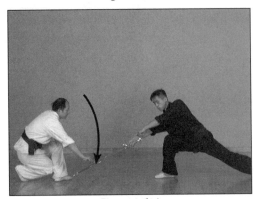

Figure 5-61A

Figure 5-60: Move the left leg west into the false stance as the sword tip travels up and then forward in a circular motion to the position shown. The left hand points forward to the west.

Figure 5-61: Change the stance into the unicorn stance, left leg forward, as the sword moves down with the tip pointing left to the south. The left hand returns to the right wrist; the right palm is down.

Figure 5-61A: White covers Black's attack straight down.

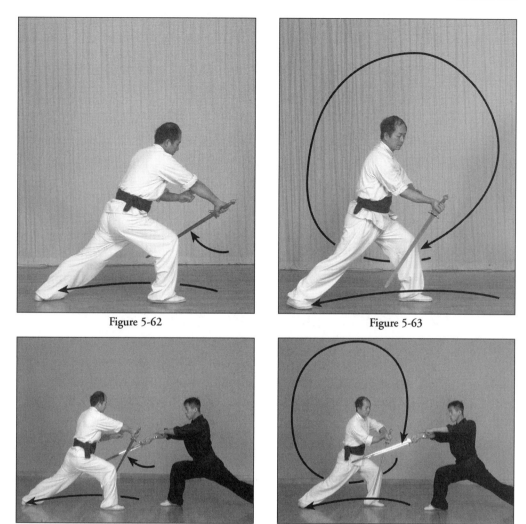

Figure 5-62

Figure 5-63

Figure 5-62A

Figure 5-63A

Figure 5-62: Step back to the east with the left leg into the bow and arrow stance, right leg forward, as the sword tip moves to the rear and the upper body twists to the left.

Figure 5-62A: White steps back and guides Black's attack to the side.

Figure 5-63: Move the right leg back into the bow and arrow stance with the left leg forward. At the same time rotate the right wrist clockwise so that the sword tip travels up, forward, down, and then to the right rear. The body is twisted to the right.

Figure 5-63A: White steps back and guides Black's attack to the side.

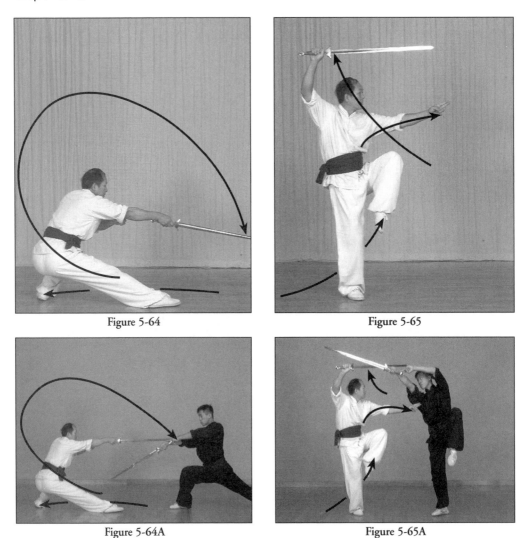

Figure 5-64

Figure 5-65

Figure 5-64A

Figure 5-65A

Figure 5-64: Step back to the east with the left leg into the taming the tiger stance, and bring the sword tip over the head and chop down to the position shown.

Figure 5-64A: After blocking in Figure 5-63A, White continues his motion and chops down at Black's arms.

Figure 5-65: Lean forward on the right leg and then raise the left leg, as the right wrist rotates counterclockwise 180 degrees, raising the sword straight up to the position shown, with the right palm facing north. Point forward and slightly up with the left hand.

Figure 5-65A: By raising his sword, White blocks Black's attack, and attacks Black's armpit with his left hand.

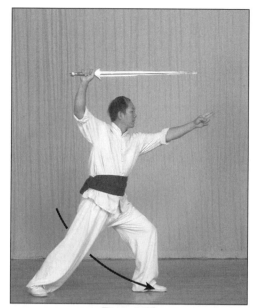

Figure 5-66

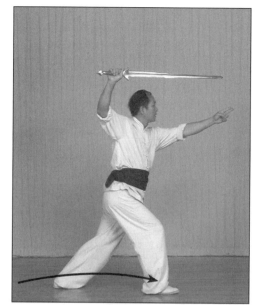

Figure 5-67

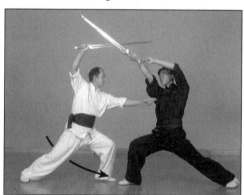

Figure 5-66A

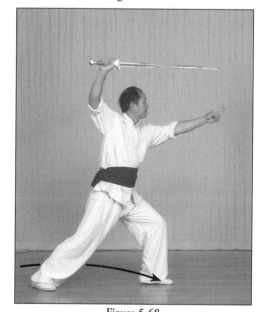

Figure 5-68

Figure 5-66: Step forward with the left leg into the bow and arrow stance.

Figure 5-66A: White follows Black's retreat.

Figure 5-67: Step forward with the right leg into the unicorn stance.

Figures 5-68 and 5-69: Repeat Figures 5-66 and 5-67.

219

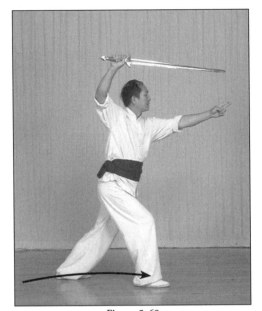

Figure 5-69

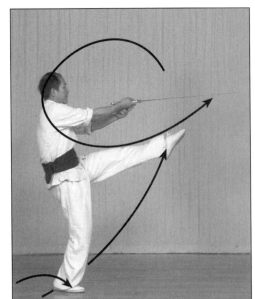

Figure 5-71

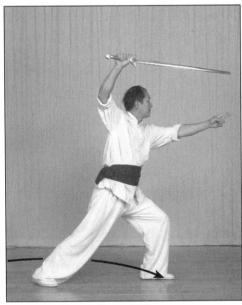

Figure 5-70

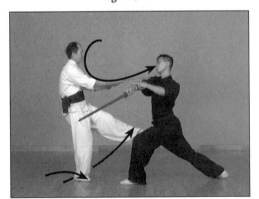

Figure 5-71A

Figure 5-70: Repeat Figure 5-66.

Figure 5-71: Step forward with the right foot. After you raise the right leg, spring off the left foot and kick with the left foot. While kicking, swing the sword in a horizontal circle from right to left to the position shown. The left hand moves to the right wrist.

Figure 5-71A: White's horizontal motion with the sword blocks Black's sword as White cuts Black's neck and kicks his groin.

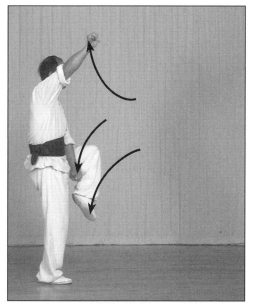

Figure 5-72

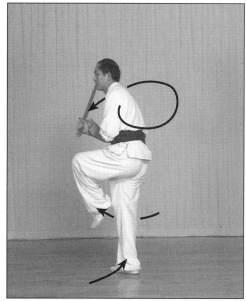

Figure 5-73

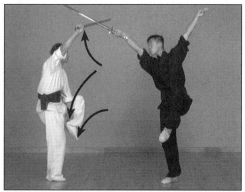

Figure 5-72A

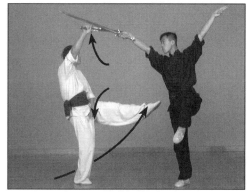

Figure 5-72B

Figure 5-72: Bring the left foot back to the position shown as the left hand, palm down, moves in front of the groin, and raise the sword up with the tip pointing to the left (south). The body faces west.

Figure 5-72A: White blocks Black's chop down to his head.

Figure 5-72B: By keeping his foot up, White keeps his option of kicking Black.

Figures 5-73 and 5-74: Jump up and turn the body 180 degrees to the left in the air and land on the left foot. At the same time, move the sword handle to the abdomen with the sword pointing south and up. The left hand returns to the right wrist. The body faces east.

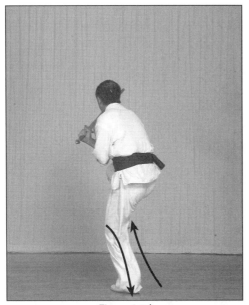

Figure 5-74

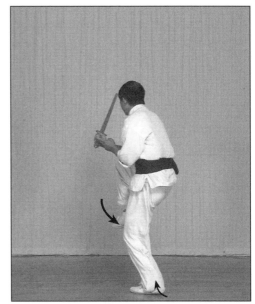

Figure 5-75

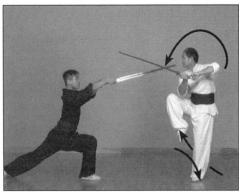

Figure 5-74A

Figure 5-74A: By dropping the sword handle and turning the trunk, White blocks Black's attack to the side.

Figures 5-75 and 5-76: Jump up again slightly off the left foot and change the position of the feet as the left foot is now raised. As the right foot lands, thrust the sword to the right, palm up, with the left hand pointing in the opposite direction.

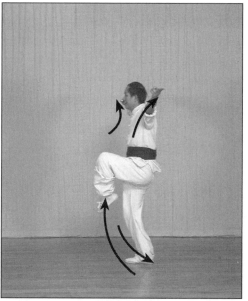

Figure 5-76

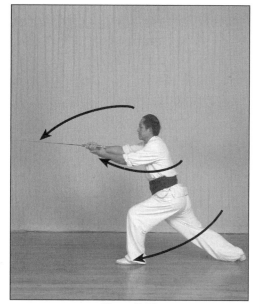

Figure 5-77

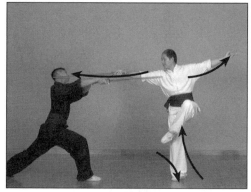

Figure 5-76A

Figure 5-76A: After blocking in Figure 5-74A, White thrusts his sword toward Black.

Figure 5-77: Step down and forward to the east with the left leg into the bow and arrow stance and swing the sword horizontally from right to left at the same time, ending with the sword in front of the body with the left hand on the right wrist. Right palm faces upward.

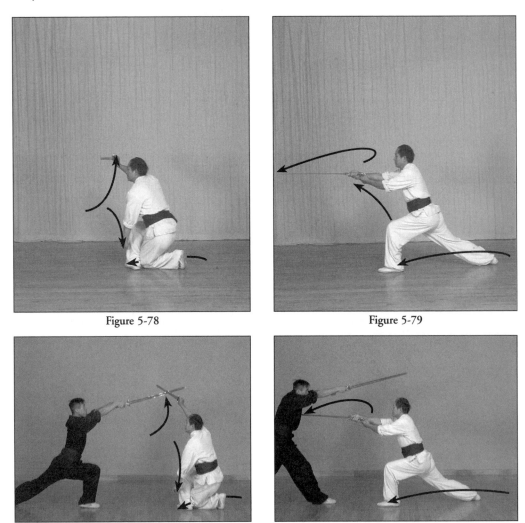

Figure 5-78

Figure 5-79

Figure 5-78A

Figure 5-79A

Figure 5-78: Step forward to the east with the right foot into the unicorn stance, moving the sword arm straight up with the tip pointing to the left, and moving the left hand down to the position shown, pointing to the right.

Figure 5-78A: White guides Black's sword up and over his head.

Figure 5-79: Step forward with the left leg into the bow and arrow stance and swing the sword horizontally from right to left at the same time, ending with the sword in front of the body with the left hand on the right wrist. Right palm faces upward.

Figure 5-79A: After blocking in Figure 5-78A, White steps in and cuts Black's midsection.

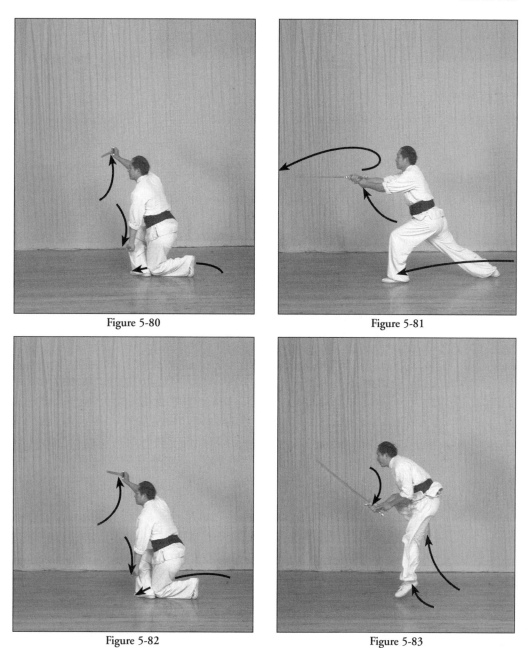

Figure 5-80

Figure 5-81

Figure 5-82

Figure 5-83

Figures 5-80 to 5-82: Repeat Figures 5-78, 5-79 and then 5-78 again.

Figures 5-83 and 5-84: Raise the left leg, and then jump up and land on it, leaving the right leg up in the position shown, and drop the sword handle as shown. The left hand moves to the right wrist.

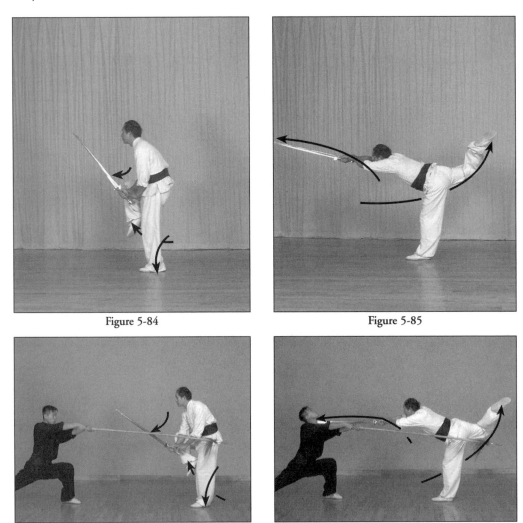

Figure 5-84

Figure 5-85

Figure 5-84A

Figure 5-85A

Figure 5-84A: White drops the sword handle down and uses this motion to help guide Black's weapon to the side.

Figure 5-85: Continuing this motion, thrust the sword forward, and at the same time, move the right leg back in mid-air. The right palm faces north.

Figure 5-85A: After blocking in Figure 5-84A, White extends his arms as far as possible to attack Black and extends his leg for balance.

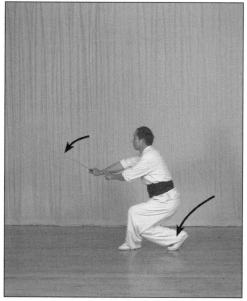

Figure 5-86

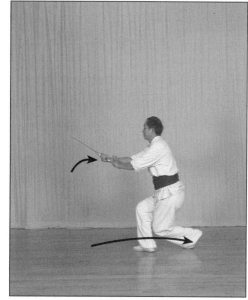

Figure 5-87

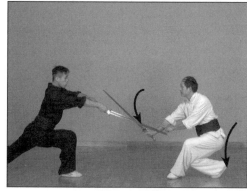

Figure 5-86A

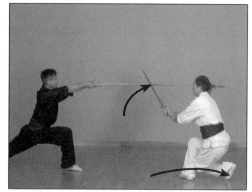

Figure 5-87A

Figure 5-86: Step down to the west with the right foot into the unicorn stance and begin shifting the weight to that leg as the right wrist rotates 90 degrees counterclockwise until the right palm faces down. The sword tip travels in a 90 degree arc to the left.

Figure 5-86A: White covers Black's sword to the left by rotating his hand counterclockwise.

Figure 5-87: Step back to the west with the left leg into the unicorn stance and rotate the right wrist clockwise 180 degrees, ending with the right palm upward. The sword tip travels in a 180 degree arc to the right.

Figure 5-87A: White guides Black's attack to the right.

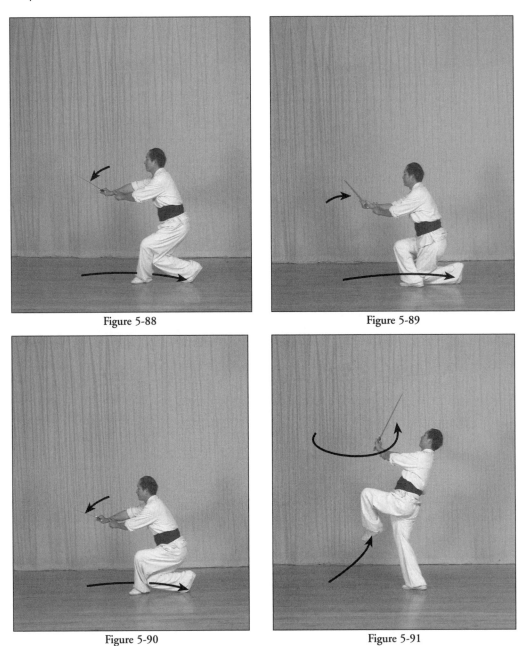

Figure 5-88

Figure 5-89

Figure 5-90

Figure 5-91

Figures 5-88 to 5-90: Repeat Figures 5-86, 5-87, and then 5-86 again.

Figure 5-91: Raise the left leg and lean back. At the same time rotate the right wrist as the sword tip travels down, to the left, and then up and to the right in front of the face.

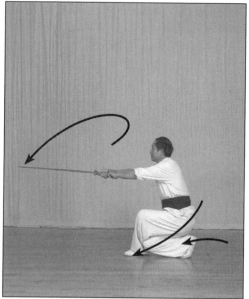

Figure 5-92

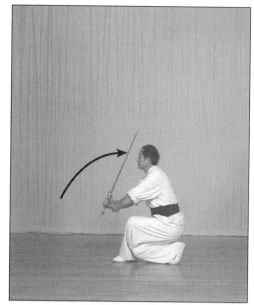

Figure 5-93

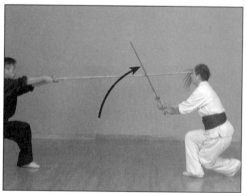

Figure 5-93A

Figure 5-92: Step down with the left foot into the unicorn stance (left leg forward), and thrust the sword forward as shown with the right palm facing upward.

Figure 5-93: Keeping the same stance, lower the sword handle and withdraw the sword tip toward you and to the right.

Figure 5-93A: White guides Black's weapon away and to the right.

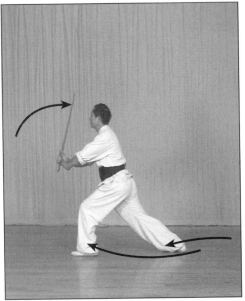

Figure 5-94

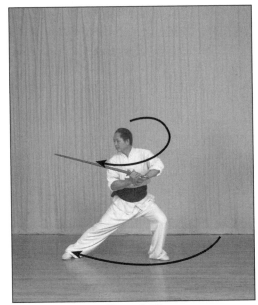

Figure 5-95

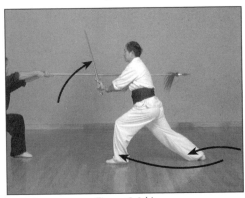

Figure 5-94A

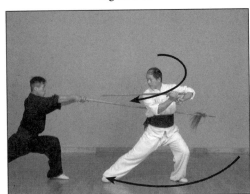

Figure 5-95A

Figure 5-94: Keeping the same arm position, step forward with the left leg into the bow and arrow stance.

Figure 5-94A: White uses his sword to keep Black's weapon away from him as he approaches Black.

Figure 5-95: Turning 180 degrees to the right, step east with the right foot. The arms stay in the same position.

Figure 5-95A: After blocking Black's attack, White turns right and steps backward to approach Black.

Figure 5-96: Step to the east with the left leg, behind the right, so that the left foot touches with the toes only. As this last step occurs, thrust the sword to the east and slightly down. The left hand points in the opposite direction from the sword.

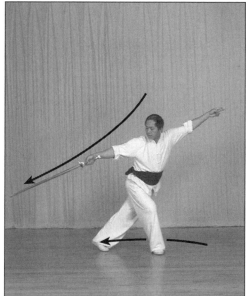

Figure 5-96

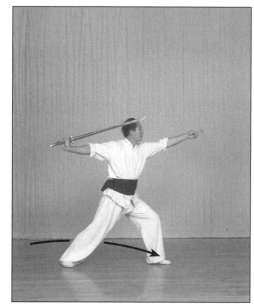

Figure 5-98

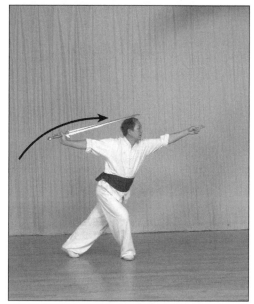
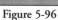

Figure 5-97

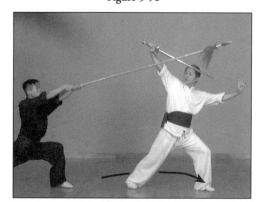

Figure 5-98A

Figure 5-97: Keeping the same stance, twist the upper body slightly to the left to face west, and rotate the right wrist counterclockwise, causing the sword tip to travel in a vertical half circle from east to west, ending in the position shown.

Figure 5-98: Keeping the same position, step forward to the west with the left leg into the bow and arrow stance.

Figure 5-98A: White wards off Black's weapon.

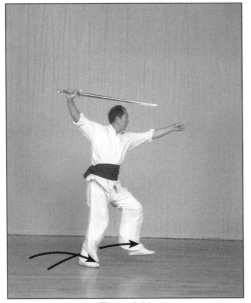

Figure 5-99

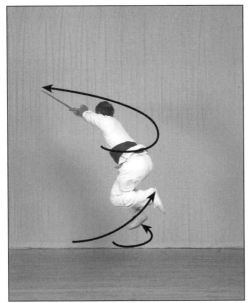

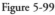

Figure 5-100

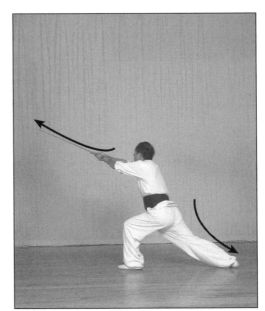

Figure 5-101

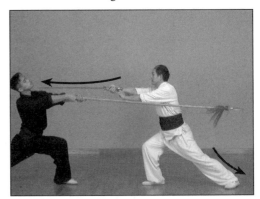

Figure 5-101A

Figure 5-99: Continuing the forward motion, raise the right foot slightly off the ground, and then quickly stomp down with it as the left foot leaves the ground. When the left foot touches the ground again, jump high and forward by springing off the left leg.

Figures 5-100 and 5-101: While still in the air, begin rotating the body to the left to face southeast, and land on the right foot. The right foot lands to the northwest of the right, and the chest faces southeast. As the right foot lands, thrust the sword forward and slightly up with the left hand returning to the right wrist. The right palm faces up, and the left leg is raised for balance.

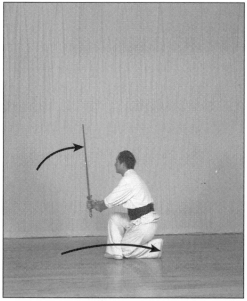

Figure 5-102

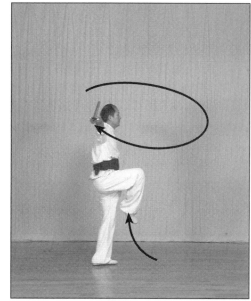

Figure 5-103

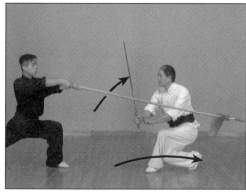

Figure 5-102A

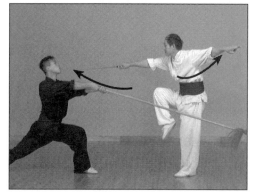

Figure 5-103A

Figure 5-101A: White avoids Black's attack by jumping to the side, and then attacks.

Figure 5-102: Step back to the west with the right leg into the unicorn stance, left leg forward. At the same time, lower the sword handle until the blade is vertical.

Figure 5-102A: White guides Black's weapon to the rear and left.

Figure 5-103: Stand straight up, raise the right leg, and spin the body 180 degrees to the right on the left foot. During this spin, swing the sword horizontally from left to right, and the left hand from right to left, ending in the position shown, with both palms facing down. The chest now faces west.

Figure 5-103A: After blocking Black's weapon to the side in Figure 5-102A, White cuts Black's neck.

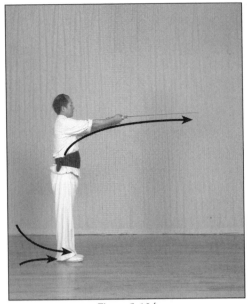

Figure 5-104

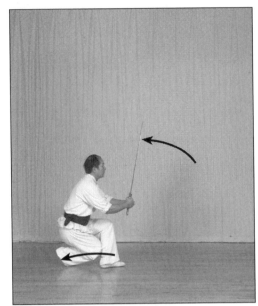

Figure 5-105

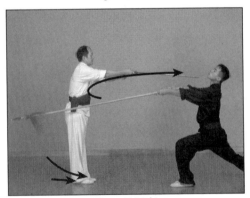

Figure 5-104A

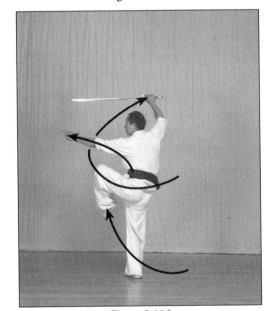

Figure 5-106

Figure 5-104: Step down and forward to the west with the right foot and lower the sword to the waist, while moving the left hand to the right wrist. Then step the left foot forward next to the right, continuing the same motion, and thrust the sword forward, palm facing upward.

Figure 5-104A: If Black withdraws and escapes the attack in Figure 5-103A, White steps toward Black and stabs his throat.

Figure 5-105: Step back with the right leg and sit down into the unicorn stance while lowering the sword hand until the blade stands vertically.

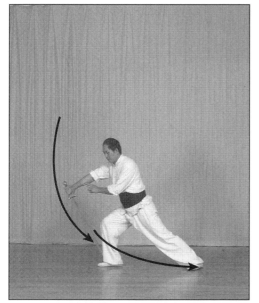

Figure 5-107

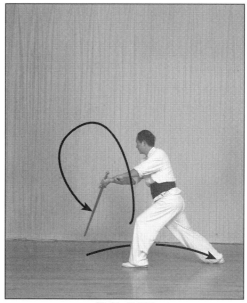

Figure 5-108

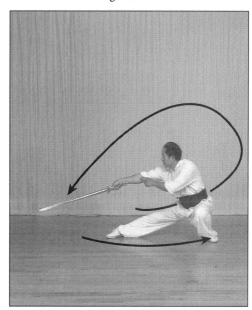

Figure 5-109

Figure 5-106: Shift all the weight to the right leg as the body spins on the right foot 180 degrees to the right, and raise the left leg to the position shown. While spinning, move the sword handle in a vertical circle so that it travels to the rear and then up over the head. The left hand moves to point forward to the east.

Figures 5-107 to 5-109: Repeat Figures 5-62 to 5-64.

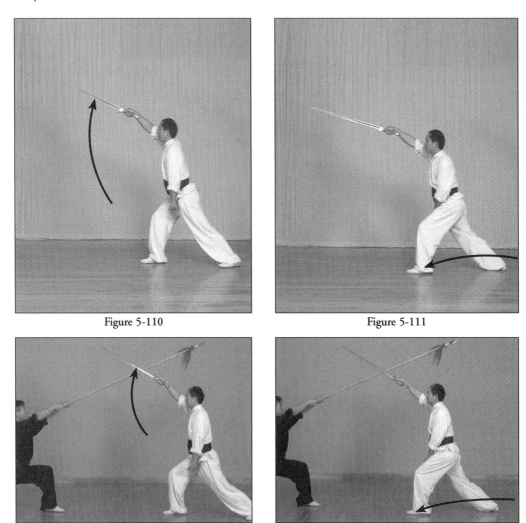

Figure 5-110

Figure 5-111

Figure 5-110A

Figure 5-111A

Figure 5-110: Shift the stance to the bow and arrow stance with the right leg forward and raise the sword to the position shown, keeping the left hand in front of the groin.

Figure 5-110A: White guides Black's weapon upward.

Figure 5-111: Keeping the same form, step forward to the east with the left leg.

Figure 5-111A: After blocking Black's weapon up, White steps in toward Black.

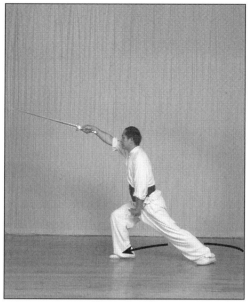

Figure 5-112

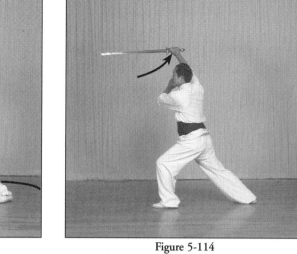

Figure 5-114

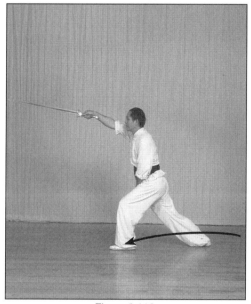

Figure 5-113

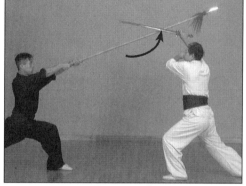

Figure 5-114A

Figures 5-112 and 5-113: Repeat Figures 5-110 and 5-111.

Figure 5-114: Lift and rotate the right hand counterclockwise and move the left hand to the right arm.

Figure 5-114A: White chases Black as he withdrew. Finally, he slides Black's weapon to the right.

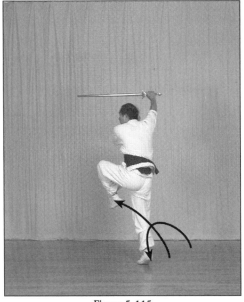

Figure 5-115

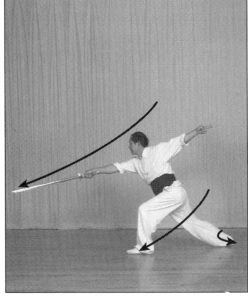

Figure 5-116

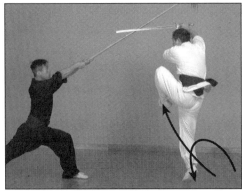

Figure 5-115A

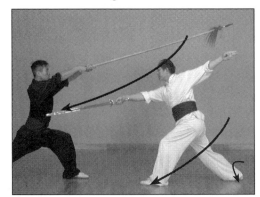

Figure 5-116A

Figure 5-115: Jump high and forward, springing off with the left foot.

Figure 5-115A: As Black retreats, White jumps toward him to gain ground.

Figure 5-116: Land on the right foot first, then the left in the bow and arrow stance while thrusting the sword forward. Point the left hand in the opposite direction.

Figure 5-116A: Finally getting within range, White stabs Black.

Figure 5-117: Shift all the weight to the left leg and raise the right foot up slightly and rotate the body 180 degrees to the left by spinning on the left foot. As the body is spinning, jump straight up by springing off the left foot. At the same time rotate the right wrist so the sword tip travels down, to the left, and then up and to the right in front of the face. The chest faces west.

Figure 5-118: As the right foot lands, kick forward with the left foot and continue the circular horizontal motion of the sword. The sword ends up pointing forward

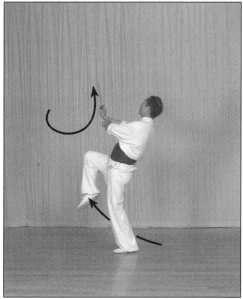

Figure 5-117

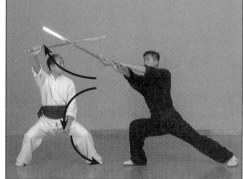

Figure 5-119

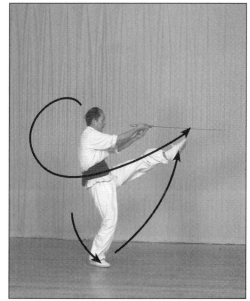

Figure 5-118

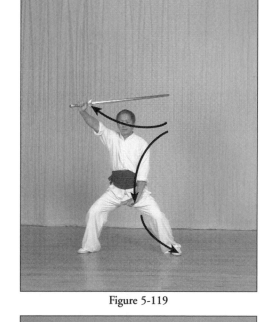

Figure 5-119A

to the west with the right palm facing upward.

Figure 5-119: Step down and forward (west) with the left leg and turn 90 degrees to the right into the horse stance. At the same time raise the sword arm so that the point remains pointing east, and move the left hand down in front of the groin. The chest faces north.

Figure 5-119A: White simply guides Black's sword up with an upward block.

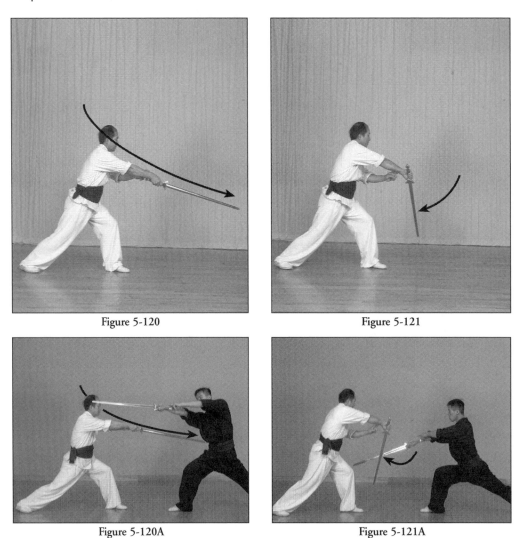

Figure 5-120

Figure 5-121

Figure 5-120A

Figure 5-121A

Figure 5-120: Twist the body 90 degrees to the left to face west in the bow and arrow stance. As the body turns, thrust the sword forward, the left hand touching the right wrist.

Figure 5-120A: After blocking in Figure 5-119A, White stabs Black's midsection.

Figure 5-121: Lower the tip of the sword to the left rear and twist the body to the left.

Figure 5-121A: White guides Black's attack away and to the left.

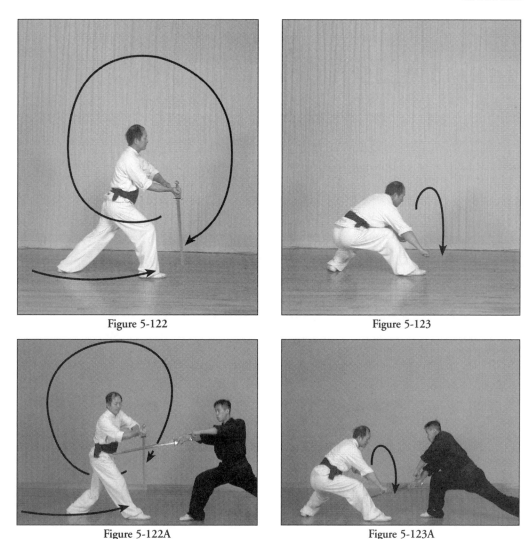

Figure 5-122

Figure 5-123

Figure 5-122A

Figure 5-123A

Figure 5-122: Without stopping, step forward to the west with the right leg and rotate the right hand 360 degrees clockwise, moving the sword tip in a clockwise circle, ending in the position shown, with the right palm facing north.

Figure 5-122A: White guides Black's attack to the side.

Figure 5-123: Continue this motion to complete a figure eight, bringing the sword tip in a counterclockwise direction up to the left, forward, and then down near the floor, and sit down into the four-six stance. The sword points southwest and the right palm faces downward.

Figure 5-123A: White's sword makes a circle and presses Black's sword down.

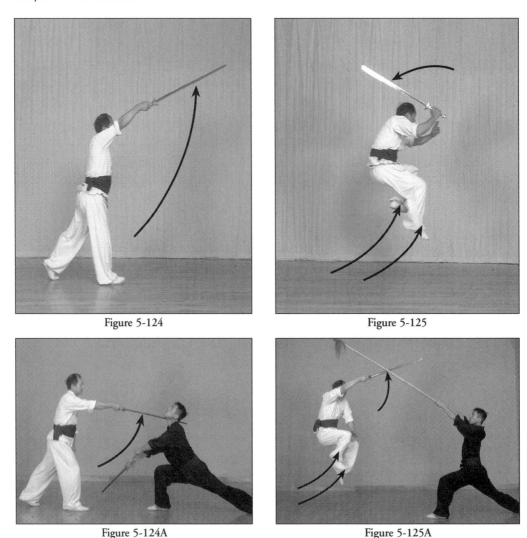

Figure 5-124

Figure 5-125

Figure 5-124A

Figure 5-125A

Figure 5-124: Rotate the right wrist clockwise while standing erect on the right leg, touching with the left toes only. As you stand, raise the sword at an angle from left to right, and move the left hand in front of the groin.

Figure 5-124A: After pressing in Figure 5-123A, White stands and leans forward to cut Black's neck, palm facing upward.

Figure 5-125: Raise the left foot slightly and then jump up and forward by springing off the right foot. While jumping, withdraw the tip of the sword toward the body until the blade stands vertical, and move the left hand to the right wrist.

Figure 5-125A: White guides Black's attack away and to the side while jumping forward.

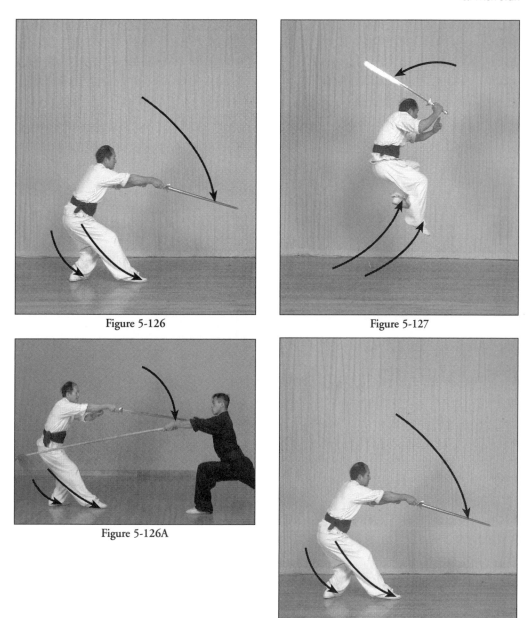

Figure 5-126

Figure 5-127

Figure 5-126A

Figure 5-128

Figure 5-126: Land on the left foot first, then step forward with the right into the false stance. At the same time, chop down with the sword to the position shown.

Figure 5-126A: After blocking in Figure 5-125A, White chops down at Black's arms.

Figures 5-127 to 5-130: Repeat Figures 5-125 and 5-126 twice.

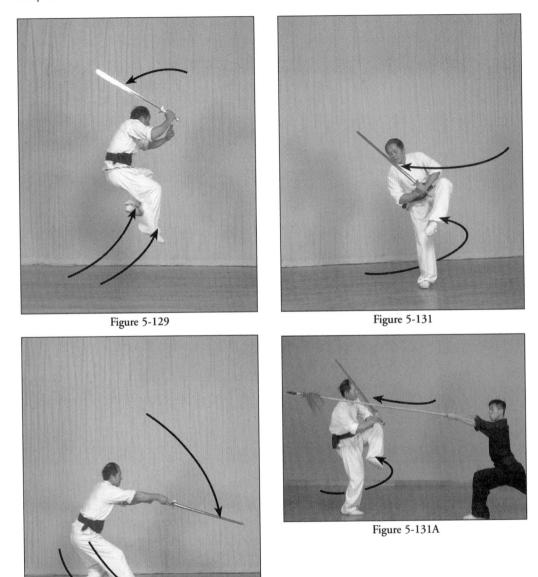

Figure 5-129

Figure 5-131

Figure 5-130

Figure 5-131A

Figures 5-131 and 5-132: Shift all the weight to the right leg as you bring the sword blade toward the right shoulder and raise the left leg. Then, spin to the right 180 degrees on the right foot.

Figures 5-131A and 5-132A: By bringing the blade in, White guides Black's weapon away and to the right. Then he spins to the right to approach Black.

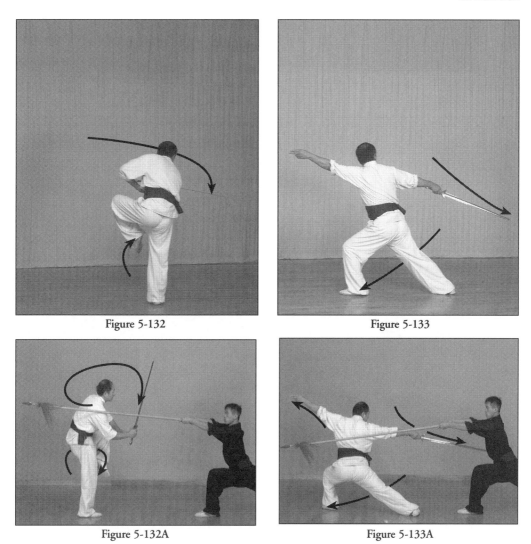

Figure 5-132

Figure 5-133

Figure 5-132A

Figure 5-133A

Figure 5-133A: By spinning, White warded off Black's weapon with his sword and opened Black up for an attack to the stomach.

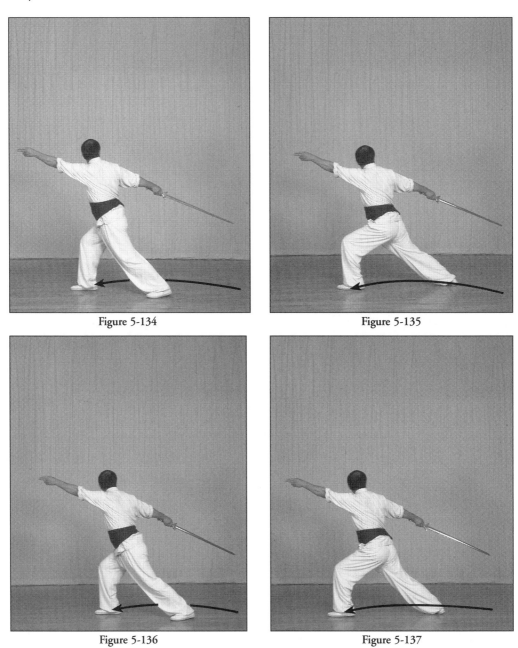

Figure 5-134

Figure 5-135

Figure 5-136

Figure 5-137

Figures 5-134 to 5-137: Take four steps forward to the east, beginning with the right leg.

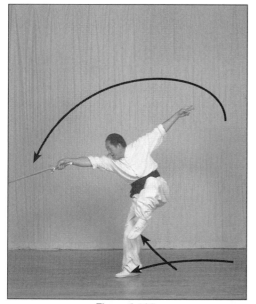

Figure 5-138

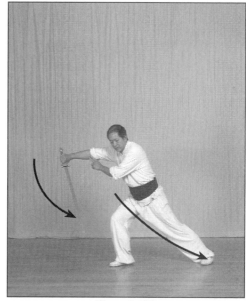

Figure 5-139

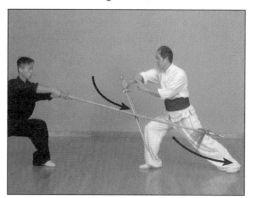

Figure 5-139A

Figure 5-138: Step again with the right leg, but this time bring both hands to the chest and thrust the sword forward and slightly down as the left foot rises to the position shown. As the sword is thrust out, the left hand extends in the opposite direction.

Figure 5-139: Step back to the west with the left leg and bring both hands together while moving the tip of the sword down slightly to the position shown.

Figure 5-139A: White guides Black's weapon away and to the left.

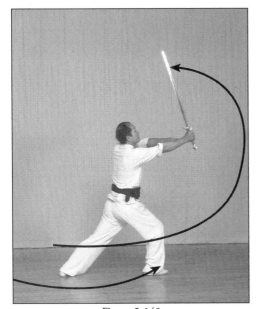

Figure 5-140

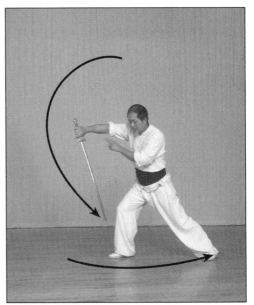

Figure 5-141

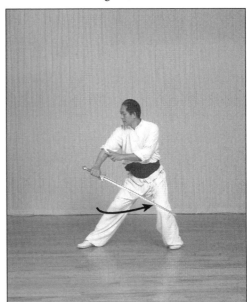

Figure 5-142

Figure 5-140: Continue to circle the sword vertically so the tip travels west, up, and then to the right over the head while stepping to the west with the right leg into the bow and arrow stance. The chest faces west and the right palm faces south.

Figure 5-141: Continue to circle the sword vertically so the tip travels up and then east while stepping the left leg west behind the right leg.

Figure 5-142: Continue to circle the sword vertically so the tip travels down, and then west while changing the stance into the four-six stance.

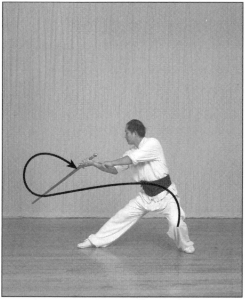

Figure 5-143

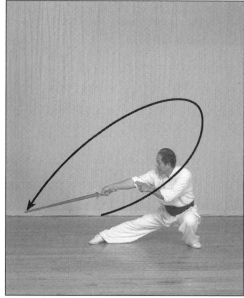

Figure 5-144

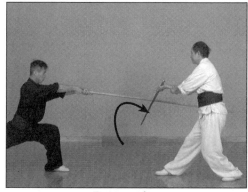

Figure 5-143A

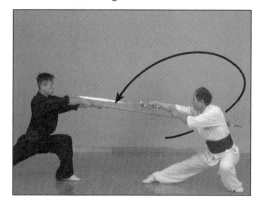

Figure 5-144A

Figure 5-143: Continue the circular motion with the sword so the tip travels in a low clockwise semicircle across the body as the body turns to face south.

Figure 5-143A: White guides Black's sword away and to the right.

Figure 5-144: Sit back on the left leg into the taming the tiger stance as shown, and bring the sword tip over the head and chop down to the position shown.

Figure 5-144A: After blocking in Figure 5-143A, White chops down at Black's arms.

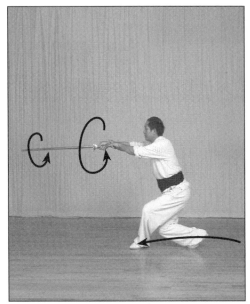

Figure 5-145

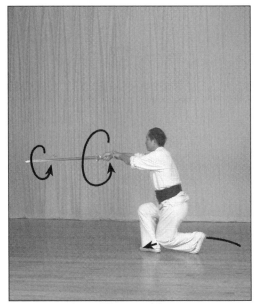

Figure 5-146

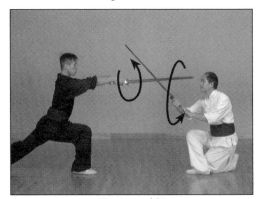

Figure 5-146A

Figure 5-145: Shift forward and step with the left leg into the unicorn stance and raise the sword to the position shown. Move the sword in a counterclockwise circular motion.

Figure 5-146: Step forward to the east with the right leg into the unicorn stance and circle the sword handle counterclockwise again.

Figure 5-146A: White moves the handle of his sword in a counterclockwise circle to block Black's attack.

Figure 5-147: Repeat Figure 5-145.

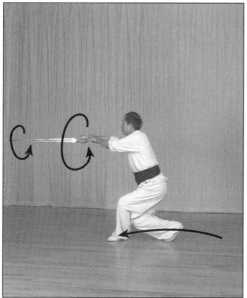

Figure 5-147

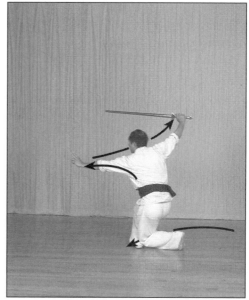

Figure 5-148

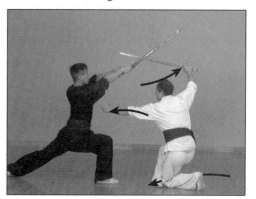

Figure 5-148A

Figure 5-148: Step forward with the right leg into the crossed leg stance while moving the sword to the west on the right side of the body and moving the left hand forward.

Figure 5-148A: White guides Black's sword away and to the right with his sword.

Figure 5-149: Stand still and kick with the heel to the east.

Figure 5-149A: White blocks Black's arms with his left hand as he kicks Black's chest.

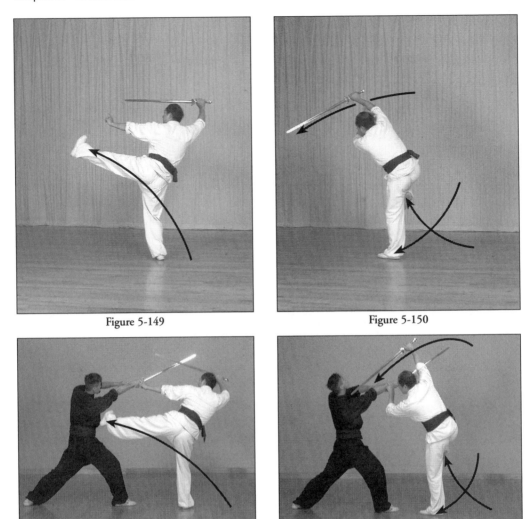

Figure 5-149

Figure 5-150

Figure 5-149A

Figure 5-150A

Figure 5-150: Step down and forward to the east with the left leg, and then raise the right leg and stab the sword from over the head down slightly to the east while returning the left hand to the right arm. The upper body also leans to the east.

Figure 5-150A: After covering Black's arm with his left hand, White stabs down at Black's throat.

Figures 5-151 and 5-152: Jump up off the left foot and turn the body 180 degrees to the left while in the air to face west. At the same time the sword makes a clockwise circle in front of the face and the upper body leans back. Just as you land on your right foot, kick with your left foot to the west and continue to circle the sword horizontally until it points west. The right palm faces upward. These two figures are the same as Figures 5-117 and 5-118.

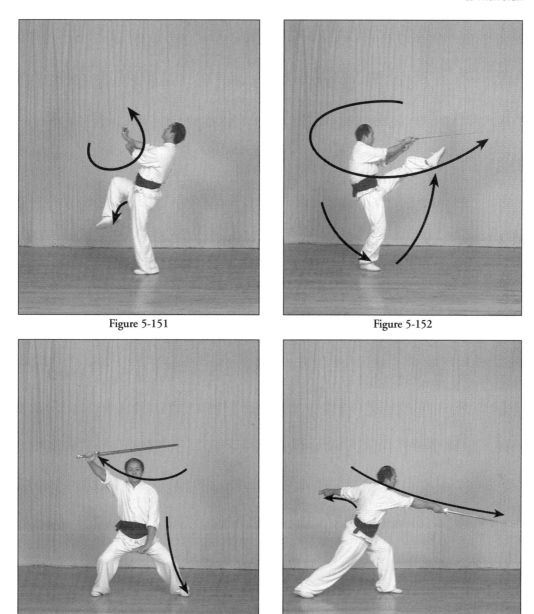

Figure 5-151

Figure 5-152

Figure 5-153

Figure 5-154

Figure 5-153: Step down and forward to the west with the left leg and turn 90 degrees to the right into the horse stance. At the same time raise the sword arm so that the point remains pointing west, and move the left hand down in front of the groin. The chest faces north.

Figure 5-154: Twist the body 90 degrees to the left to face west into the bow and arrow stance. As the body turns, thrust the sword forward, pointing the left hand in the opposite direction.

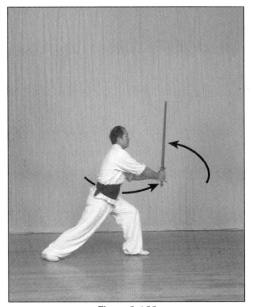

Figure 5-155

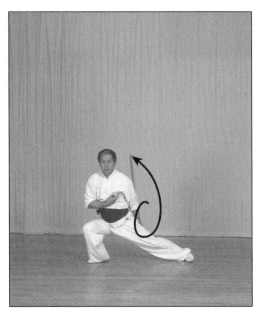

Figure 5-156

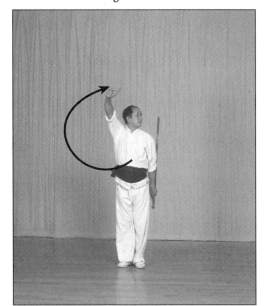

Figure 5-157

Figure 5-155: Rotate the right wrist clockwise so that the tip of the sword travels down, to the left, and then up to the position shown. The left hand is palm up with the sword handle between the thumb and first finger.

Figure 5-156: Grasp the sword with the left hand and circle the sword tip clockwise in a 360 degree circle in a north-south plane. The right hand moves to the midsection.

Figure 5-157: Bring the left foot back next to the right and stand upright facing north. At the same time move the sword next to the body and circle the right hand smoothly from the waist down, to the right, up, and then to the left over the head to the position shown.

CHAPTER 6

Free Fighting Training and Strategy

自由對練與戰策

6-1. INTRODUCTION

Learning to fight with a sword is like learning to fight barehanded. The student begins by learning set fighting forms, practices them with a partner, and then moves to free fighting. The forms must be practiced until the reactions are natural. In order to keep from acquiring bad habits, the student should only begin free fighting after he is familiar with all the fighting forms. In the beginning of two-person practice, keep a safe distance from each other and concentrate attacks on the wrists and arms. Use wooden swords for safety, and move slowly, letting speed and power come of their own accord. The reader should understand that the fighting forms and free fighting training procedures presented here are typical examples, and that there are many others in existence. The forms and techniques presented here will give the student a proper start in this training. After he has become familiar with all the techniques presented, the student will be able to research and develop additional techniques, and to create his own forms, suited to his own needs.

6-2. FIGHTING FORMS

Many fighting forms can be extracted from the solo sequences presented in the previous chapters. Forms that are good for training must be continuous, repeatable defensive and offensive techniques. The main purpose of a fighting form is to make the reactions natural. Here, fifteen examples of fighting forms will be presented in four sets: straight line attack and defense, right side attack and defense, left side attack and defense, and then continuous forms.

Straight Line Attack and Defense.

These forms should be practiced as a back and forth exchange. First one partner attacks and the other defends, then the other partner executes the same tack and the first defends the same way.

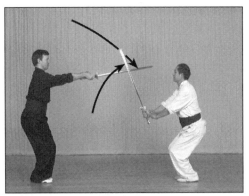

Figure 6-1

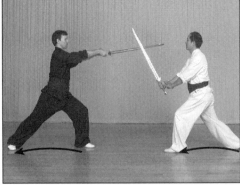

Figure 6-2

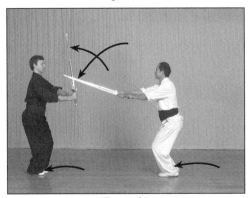

Figure 6-3

Form 1 (Figures 6-1 to 6-3). Black stabs at White, who steps back and blocks up and to the right, then steps forward and slide cuts down to Black's arm or wrist. Black steps backward and blocks this thrust the same way and repeats the attack.

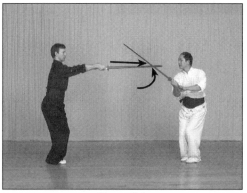

Figure 6-4

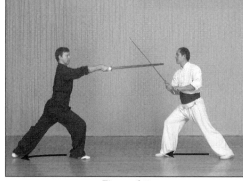

Figure 6-5

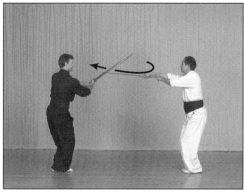

Figure 6-6

Form 2 (Figures 6-4 to 6-6). Black stabs at White with right palm facing downward. White blocks by deflecting Black's sword to the left, then steps forward and stabs at Black's throat. Black steps backward and blocks this thrust the same way and repeats the attack.

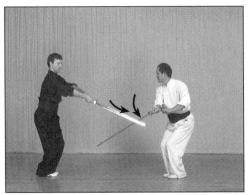

Figure 6-7

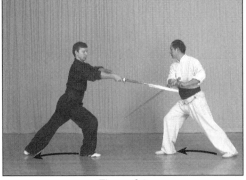

Figure 6-8

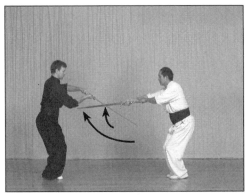

Figure 6-9

Form 3 (Figures 6-7 to 6-9). Black stabs at White's stomach. White steps backward and deflects Black's sword down to the left, then steps forward and stabs toward Black's stomach. Black steps backward and blocks this thrust the same way and repeats the attack.

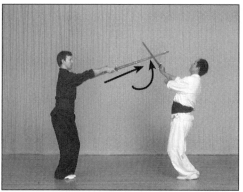

Figure 6-10

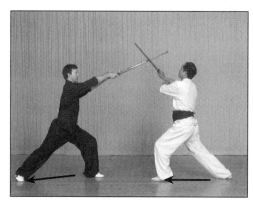

Figure 6-11

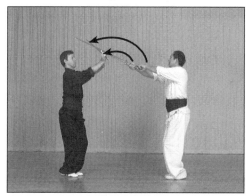

Figure 6-12

Form 4 (Figures 6-10 to 6-12). Black stabs at White's face. White blocks by deflecting Black's sword to the right while leaning backward, then steps forward and stabs at Black's face. Black steps backward and blocks this thrust the same way and repeats the attack.

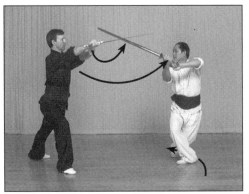

Figure 6-13

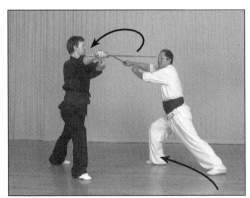

Figure 6-14

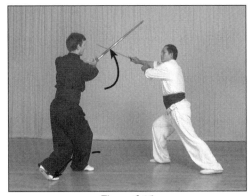

Figure 6-15

Right Side Attack and Defense

Form 5 (Figures 6-13 to 6-15). Black stabs at White's head from his right side. White blocks by stepping to the right by moving his left foot behind his right and deflecting Black's sword up and to the left. He then steps forward with his right foot into the bow and arrow stance and stabs at Black's head from his right. Black blocks this thrust the same way and repeats the attack.

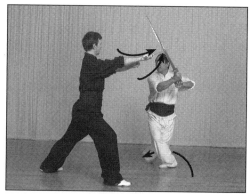

Figure 6-16

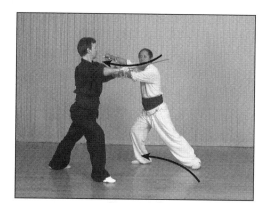

Figure 6-17

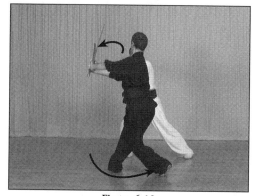

Figure 6-18

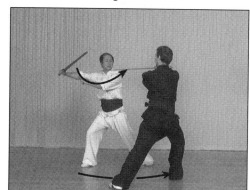

Figure 6-19

Form 6 (Figures 6-16 to 6-19). Black cuts at White's neck. White blocks by stepping to the right by moving his left foot behind his right and deflecting Black's sword up and to the left, then steps forward with his right foot into the bow and arrow stance and cuts at Black's neck. Black blocks the same way and repeats the attack.

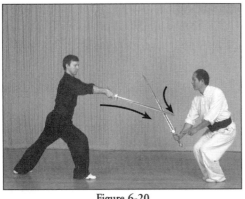

Figure 6-20

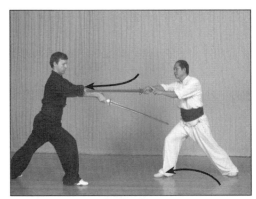

Figure 6-21

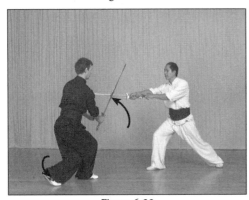

Figure 6-22

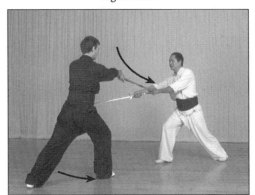

Figure 6-23

Form 7 (Figures 6-20 to 6-23). Black slides and cuts at White's wrist. White blocks by stepping to the right by moving his left foot behind his right and deflecting Black's sword to the left, then steps forward with his right foot into the bow and arrow stance and slide cuts at Black's wrist. Black blocks the same way and repeats the attack.

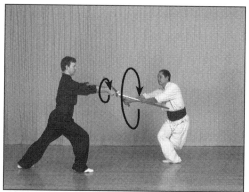

Figure 6-24

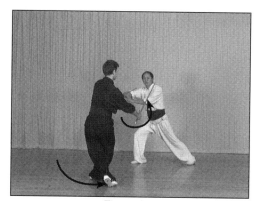

Figure 6-25

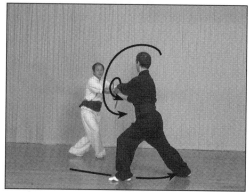

Figure 6-26

Form 8 (Figures 6-24 to 6-26). White cuts right to left down at Black's wrist from the outside. Black counters by stepping to the right by moving his left foot behind his right. At the same time, he evades White's sword by moving his wrist counterclockwise from under the sword and bringing his own sword higher than White's. He then steps forward with his right foot into the bow and arrow stance and cuts at White's wrist. White blocks the same way and repeats the attack. This form is called Sword Wrap Hand. It is performed continuously with the partners circling each other.

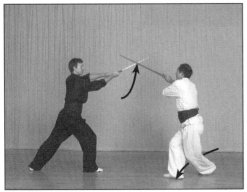

Figure 6-27

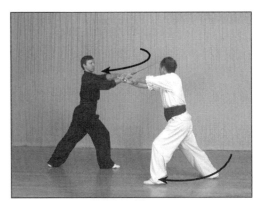

Figure 6-28

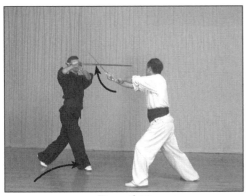

Figure 6-29

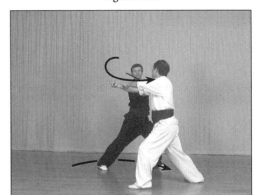

Figure 6-30

Left Side Attack and Defense

Form 9 (Figures 6-27 to 6-30). Black cuts at White's neck. White steps to the left, moving his right leg in front of his left, and at the same time deflects Black's sword to the right by raising his sword to vertical. White then moves into a bow and arrow stance with his left leg and cuts at Black's neck. Black blocks this cut the same way and repeats the attack.

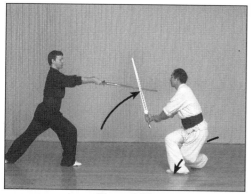

Figure 6-31

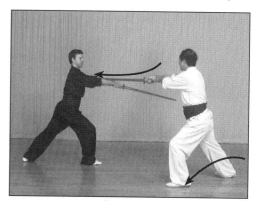

Figure 6-32

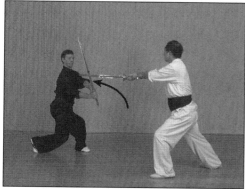

Figure 6-33

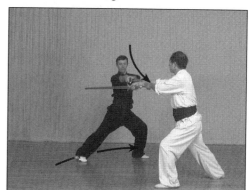

Figure 6-34

Form 10 (Figures 6-31 to 6-34). Black chops at White's wrists from the outside. White counters by stepping to the left by moving his right foot in front of his left. At the same time, he evades Black's sword by moving his wrist clockwise from under the sword and bringing his sword to Black's right side. He then steps forward with his left foot into the bow and arrow stance and cuts from right to left at Black's wrist. Black blocks the same way and repeats the chop.

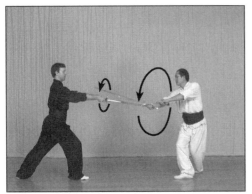

Figure 6-35

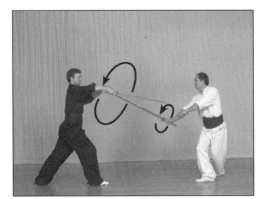

Figure 6-36

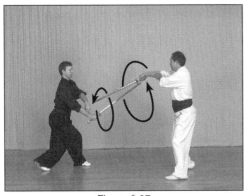

Figure 6-37

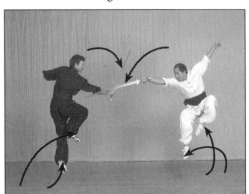

Figure 6-38

Form 11 (Figures 6-35 to 6-37). This is the left side to the Sword Wrap Hand practice presented in Form 8. In this exercise, White steps with the right leg to the left in front of the left leg and at the same time slide cuts Black's wrist. In order to avoid White's cut, Black steps with his right leg to the left in front of the left leg and at the same time raises his right wrist to the left. Black then steps forward with his left leg and slide cuts White's wrist.

Form 12 (Figure 6-38). Both Black and White jump off the left foot, lean forward, and chop at the other's sword wrist. They land on the right foot and repeat, circling each other as they repeat the jumping.

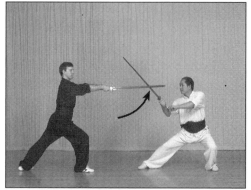

Figure 6-39

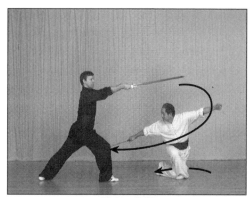

Figure 6-40

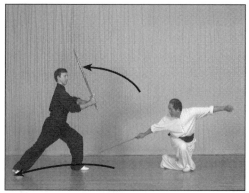

Figure 6-41

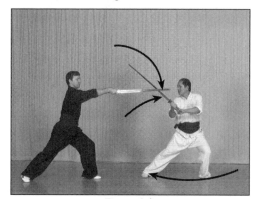

Figure 6-42

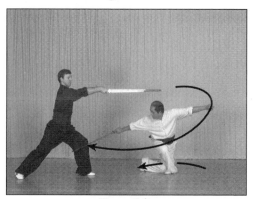

Figure 6-43

Continuous Forms

These forms are executed repeatedly in a straight line, with Black attacking and White countering. Unlike the forms above in which White and Black exchange roles continuously, White and Black keep the same roles throughout the exercise.

Form 13 (Figures 6-39 to 6-43). Black steps forward with his right foot and chops at White's head. White twists to the left and deflects the thrust up and to the left, then steps into the crossed leg stance with his left foot and cuts to Black's knee. Black steps backward and withdraws his sword, then chops at White's head again. White steps forward and blocks, then steps into the crossed leg stance and attacks. Repeat continuously.

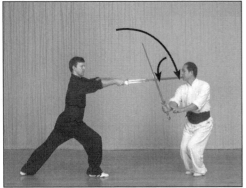

Figure 6-44

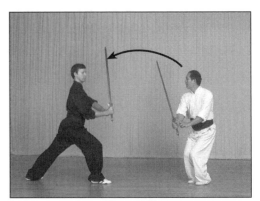

Figure 6-45

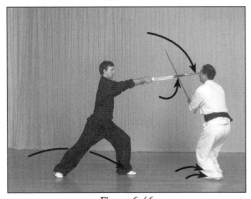

Figure 6-46

Form 14 (Figures 6-44 to 6-46). Black steps forward with his right foot and stabs at White's chest. White twists to the left and deflects the thrust to the left. Black then steps forward with his left foot and stabs at White's chest. White steps backward, twists to the right and deflects the thrust to the right. The form is then repeated continuously.

Form 15 (Figures 6-47 to 6-51). Black steps forward with his right foot and stabs at White's head. White twists to the left and deflects the thrust up and to the left, then steps into the false stance with his left foot and cuts under Black's sword to Black's chest. Black steps back with his right leg into the four-six stance, then moves forward into the bow and arrow stance, stabbing at White's head. White steps back and deflects to the left, then steps forward and cuts at Black's chest under Black's sword. Repeat continuously.

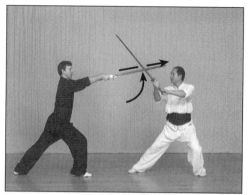

Figure 6-47

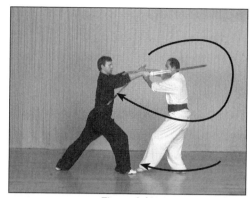

Figure 6-48

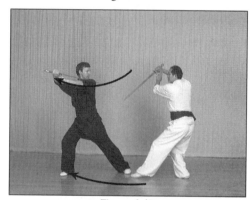

Figure 6-49

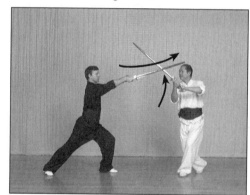

Figure 6-50

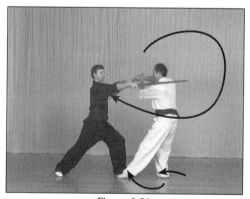

Figure 6-51

6-3. Free Fighting Training

The best sword tactic is to attack the enemy without blocking his weapon. The ability to do this shows great skill because of the economy of your movement. In addition, by not blocking you extend the life of your sword. The most important reason to use this tactic, however, is that by attacking without blocking you can injure the enemy much more easily than when you block first and then attack. This is because when your enemy is attacking you, his consciousness is focused on attacking and not on protection. In the Chinese martial arts there is a saying, "The best time to attack your enemy is while he is attacking you." Therefore, attack is the best defense. Naturally these techniques are the hardest and usually take a great deal of practice and experience before you can react with speed, power, and the right technique. The key to avoiding the enemy's attack is swift leg movement. An example of this technique is if your enemy stabs at your stomach, you step to the right to avoid the attack and at the same time stab your enemy's body.

The most common and easiest sword fighting tactic is to slide block or use the dull part of the sword to direct the enemy's attack aside, and then to counterattack. These techniques are safer and usually the right starting moves for a sword beginner. Only after you have enough experience in blocking techniques should you try to attack without blocking. The first principle of free fighting strategy is self-defense first and offense second. When you practice, always act as though the swords are razor sharp so that the slightest touch will injure you and make you lose the battle. Wooden swords should be used, but remember that even a wooden sword can sometimes cause injuries. Always treat the wooden sword as if it were a real sword.

To start free fighting training, both practitioners stand just out of sword range, facing each other with feet parallel. Then both sides attack and block. Use any of the techniques learned from the previous sections, such as chopping, stabbing, or slide cuts. If your partner attacks you, and you do not clearly neutralize the attack, then you have lost the fight. Only after both partners can block each other without hesitation or difficulty should the distance they stand from each other be shortened. At that time, begin at a distance where you can just touch each other with the sword tips.

After both practitioners can block each other's attacks at this short distance, you can start moving forward and backward while attacking and blocking. At this stage, leg movement becomes the determining factor in winning. Only when both partners can block each other without any problem should you go to the next stage.

The third stage is to incorporate dodging to the right and left, to avoid attacks or to attack your partner. Continue to practice with the techniques already learned.

When the above three stages of free fighting are mastered, with good blocking reactions, good leg movement, and effective attacking techniques, then the student is a qualified sword fighter. It usually takes at least three years of practicing three hours a day to reach this level. Using kicking and hand strikes, or grabs in coordination with the sword techniques, is a higher level of achievement that will allow you to disable an enemy at very short range, where because of its length, the sword is hard to use effectively.

CHAPTER 7

Conclusion

結論

This book has introduced the fundamental training, and three typical sequences of northern sword. However the reader should understand that in order to master the sword, he should first study and master the saber. In addition he will need a qualified master to guide him in the sword techniques. Although this book has introduced both fundamental and advanced techniques, it would be extremely hard for any martial artist to learn them just from this book. However, if a person has learned similar sword techniques from another northern style, he will be able to grasp most of the key points is this book.

Roughly speaking, a person without any previous sword training would need about two years to learn the three sequences in this book. It would then take several additional years to really master them.

The authors remind the reader that the forms and techniques in a sequence remain dead unless they can be used as natural reactions. In order to develop this, students should practice continually with partners, until all their reactions and use of the techniques become natural. Chapter Six explained this method of practice.

The last point the authors want to stress is that any practitioner who has learned only from this book should not teach the sequences. The fundamental training methods, such as exercises and stances, can be taught, but only after mastering them. Sequences are much harder to preserve accurately unless one has learned from the original source.

The reader should understand that the training is difficult and time consuming. Proficiency will come only after years of practice, and consistency of ability will come only after decades. It would not be called Gongfu if it were easy to learn and master. Patience, perseverance, and, most importantly, strength of will are the primary virtues needed to master this art. If you can demonstrate all these traits, you have learned to control your emotions, especially laziness, procrastination, and fear. Only then will you be prepared to learn what the sword has to offer. The most challenging opponent you are ever likely to meet in your sword practice is yourself. Only when you can master yourself, can you really say that you are practicing Gongfu.

Time Table of Chinese History

Chinese	English Translation	Duration
五帝紀	The Age of the Five Rulers	2852–2205 B.C. (647 Years)
夏紀	The Xia Dynasty	2205–1766 B.C. (439 Years)
商紀(殷紀)	The Shang Dynasty (or Yin Dynasty)	1766–1122 B.C. (644 Years)
周紀	The Zhou Dynasty	1122–255 B.C. (867 Years)
秦紀	The Qin dynasty	255–206 B.C. (49 Years)
漢紀(前漢)(西漢)	The Han Dynasty (Former Han or Western Han)	206 B.C.–25 A.D. (231 Years)
後漢紀	The Later Han Dynasty (Eastern Han)	25–221 A.D. (196 Years)
三國	Epoch of The Three Kingdoms	221–265 A.D.
I. 蜀漢紀	The Minor Han Dynasty	221–265 A.D. (44 Years)
II. 魏紀	The Wei Dynasty	220–265 A.D. (45 Years)
III. 吳紀	The Wu Dynasty	222–278 A.D. (56 Years)
西晉紀	The Western Jin Dynasty	265–317 A.D. (52 Years)
東晉紀	The Eastern Jin Dynasty	317–420 A.D. (103 Years)
南北朝	Epoch of Division Between North and South	420–589 A.D. (169 Years)
劉宋紀	The Song Dynasty (House of Liu)	420–479 A.D. (59 Years)
北魏紀	The Northern Wei Dynasty (House of Toba)	386–535 A.D. (149 Years)
西魏紀	The Western Wei Dynasty	535–557 A.D. (22 Years)
東魏紀	The Eastern Wei Dynasty	534–550 A.D. (16 Years)
北齊紀	The Northern Qi Dynasty	550–589 A.D. (39 Years)
北周紀	The Northern Zhou Dynasty	557–589 A.D. (32 Years)
齊紀	The Qi Dynasty	479–502 A.D. (23 Years)
梁紀	The Liang Dynasty	502–557 A.D. (55 Years)
陳紀	The Chen Dynasty	557–589 A.D. (32 Years)

隋紀	The Sui Dynasty	589–618 A.D. (29 Years)
唐紀	The Tang Dynasty	618–907 A.D. (389 Years)
五代	The Epoch of the Five Dynasties	907–960 A.D. (53 Years)
後梁紀	The Posterior Liang Dynasty	907–923 A.D. (16 Years)
後唐紀	The Posterior Tang Dynasty	923–936 A.D. (13 Years)
後晉紀	The Posterior Jin Dynasty	936–947 A.D. (11 Years)
後漢紀	The Posterior Han Dynasty	947–951 A.D. (4 Years)
後周紀	The Posterior Zhou Dynasty	951–960 A.D. (9 Years)
遼紀	The Liao Dynasty (Khitan Tartars)	907–1125 A.D. (218 Years)
西遼紀	The Western Liao Dynasty (Khitan Tartars)	1125–1169 A.D. (43 Years)
宋紀	The Song Dynasty	960–1127 A.D. (167 Years)
南宋紀	The Southern Song Dynasty	1127–1280 A.D. (153 Years)
金紀	The Jin Dynasty (Niu Zhen Tartars)	1115–1260 A.D. (145 Years)
元紀	The Yuan Dynasty (Mongols)	1206–1368 A.D. (162 Years)
明紀	The Ming Dynasty	1368–1644 A.D. (276 Years)
清紀	The Qing Dynasty	1644–1912 A.D. (268 Years)
中華民國	The Republic of China	1912 –

Translation and Glossary of Chinese Terms

Bai He 白鶴　Means "White Crane." One of the southern Chinese martial styles.

Bei Jian 北劍　Means "Northern Sword." The sword techniques and practice routines (i.e., sequences) created in the northern Chinese martial styles.

Bei Zhou (557-581 A.D.) 北周　Northern Zhou Dynasty. One of the dynasties in Chinese history.

Beng 弸　To extend or to expand. One of the basic sword techniques.

Bi Shou 比首　A dagger.

Cao-Cao 曹操　The ruler of Wei. Wei was one of the three kingdoms in The Three Kingdoms Dynasty that followed the Han Dynasty and lasted 60 years (220-280 A.D.).

Chang Chuan (Changquan) 長拳　Means "Long Range Fist." Chang Chuan includes all northern Chinese long range martial styles.

Chang Jiang (Yangtze River) 長江 (揚子江)　Literally, long river. Refers to the Yangtze river in southern China.

Changquan (Chang Chuan) 長拳　Means "Long Range Fist." Changquan includes all northern Chinese long range martial styles.

Cheng, Gin-Gsao 曾金灶　Dr. Yang, Jwing-Ming's White Crane master.

Chi Kung (Qigong) 氣功　The Gongfu of Qi, which means the study of Qi.

Chi You 蚩尤　The opponent of the Yellow Emperor (Huang Di) during the years 2697-2597 B.C.

Chin Na (Qin Na) 擒拿　Literally means "grab control." A component of Chinese martial arts which emphasizes grabbing techniques, to control your opponent's joints, in conjunction with attacking certain acupuncture cavities.

Chun Qiu (770-403 B.C.) 春秋　The Spring and Autumn Period. One of the Chinese historical periods.

Ci, 刺　Stab. One of the basic sword techniques.

Cuo 挫、錯　File. One of the basic sword techniques.

Deng Shan Bu (Gong Jian Bu) 蹬山步（弓箭步） The Mountain Climbing Stance or Bow and Arrow Stance. One of the fundamental stances in northern Chinese martial styles.

Di 地 Earth.

Dian 點 Point. One of the basic sword techniques.

Dian Xue Massages 點穴按摩 Chinese massage techniques in which the acupuncture cavities are stimulated through pressing. Dian Xue massage is also called acupressure, and is the root of Japanese Shiatsu.

Fu Hu Bu 伏虎步 Tame the Tiger Stance. One of the fundamental stances in northern Chinese martial styles.

Gai 蓋 Cover. One of the basic sword techniques.

Gan Jiang 干將 A very famous sword maker, who also named one of his best swords "Gan Jiang." His wife, Mo Xie was also a well-known sword maker during the Spring and Autumn Period (770-403 B.C.) and the Warring States Period (403-221 B.C.).

Ge 格 Block Upward.

Gong Jian Bu (Deng Shan Bu) 弓箭步（蹬山步） Bow and Arrow Stance or Mountain Climbing Stance. One of the fundamental stances trained in northern Chinese martial styles.

Gong (Kung) 功 Energy or hard work.

Gongfu (Kung Fu) 功夫 Means "energy-time." Anything that will take time and energy to learn or to accomplish is called Gongfu.

Gua 掛 To lift. One of the basic sword techniques.

Guoshu (Wushu) 國術(武術) Abbreviation of "Zhongguo Wushu," which means "Chinese Martial Techniques."

Han 漢 A Dynasty in Chinese history (206 B.C.-221 A.D.).

Han, Ching-Tang 韓慶堂 A well known Chinese martial artist, especially in Taiwan in the last forty years. Master Han is also Dr. Yang, Jwing-Ming's Long Fist Grand Master.

He Lu 闔閭 A Wu emperor who loved collecting swords.

Henan 河南省 The province in China where the Shaolin Temple is located.

Huai Nan Wan Hua Shu 淮南萬華術 *Huai Nan's Thousand Crafts,* a book on metallurgy.

Huang Di (2690-2590 B.C.) 黃帝 Huang Di, called the "Yellow Emperor" because he occupied the territory near the Yellow River.

Hunan Province 湖南省 A province near the middle of China.

Ji Xiao Xin Shu 紀效新書 *Book of Efficient Discipline.* A book written by Qi, Ji-Guang during Chinese Ming dynasty (1368-1644 A.D.).

Jian 劍 Sword.

Jian Dao 劍道 The sword way, including morality and training.

Jiao 絞 Wrap. One of the basic sword techniques.

Jie 揭 Rise. One of the basic sword techniques.

Jie 截 Intercept. One of the basic sword techniques.

Jin Ji Du Li 金雞獨立 The Golden Rooster Stands on One Leg Stance. One of the fundamental stances in northern Chinese martial arts.

Jin Race 金 Mongols.

Jin, Shao-Feng 金紹峰 Dr. Yang, Jwing-Ming's White Crane grand master.

Jing Wu Association 上海精武體育會 A very well-known Chinese martial arts organization founded by Huo, Yuan-Jia in Shanghai around 1909.

Ju Chi Jian 鋸齒劍 Means "Saw-Toothed Sword." A type of sword.

Ju Que 巨闕 One of the famous swords forged by Ou Ye Zi, during the Chinese Spring and Autumn Period (722-484 B.C.), and the Warring States Period (403-222 B.C.). It is said that this sword was so sharp that, if dipped in water, it would be withdrawn perfectly dry.

Kao Tao 高濤 Master Yang, Jwing-Ming's first Taijiquan master.

Kun Wu Jian 崑峿劍 Name of a sword. Also the name of a sword sequence that was passed down by Li, Yu-Xiang in Cang Xian, Hebei Province during the Qing Dynasty (1644-1911 A.D.).

Kung (Gong) 功 Means "energy" or "hard work."

Kung Fu (Gongfu) 功夫 Means "energy-time." Anything that will take time and energy to learn or to accomplish is called Kung Fu.

Lan 攔 Hinder or obstruct. One of the basic sword techniques.

Le 将 Draw back. One of the basic sword techniques.

Li, Cai-Ting 李彩亭 A well-known martial artist whom is considered to be the first one who passed down the well-known sword sequence, San Cai Jian, during the Qing Dynasty (1644-1911 A.D.).

Li, Mao-Ching 李茂清 Dr. Yang, Jwing-Ming's Long Fist master.

Li, Yu-Xiang 李玉祥 A well-known Chinese martial artist who first passed down the well-known sword sequence, Kun Wu Jian during Qing Dynasty (1644-1911 A.D.).

Lian Bing Shi Ji 練兵實紀 The name of a book, *Record of Practical Training of Soldiers,* written by Qi, Ji-Guang during the Ming dynasty (1368-1644 A.D.).

Liao 撩 Slide block and cut. One of the basic sword techniques.

Liu Bei 劉備 The ruler of Han. Han was one of the three kingdoms in The Three Kingdoms Dynasty.

Long Quan 龍泉 A county in Zhejiang Province that is well known for producing good weapons.

Long Quan Jian 龍泉劍 The swords produced from the Long Quan county in Zhejiang Province.

Ma Bu 馬步 Horse Stance. One of the fundamental stances in northern martial styles.

Ming Dynasty (1368-1644 A.D.) 明朝 One of the dynasties in Chinese history.

Mo 摸 Smear. One of the basic sword techniques.

Mo Xie 莫邪 A very famous sword maker, who named one of her best swords "Mo Xie." Her Husband, Gan Jiang was also a well-known sword maker during the Spring and Autumn Period (770-403 B.C.) and the Warring States Period (403-221 B.C.).

Nanking Central Guoshu Institute 南京中央國術館 A Chinese martial arts institute organized by the government around 1928.

National Taiwan University 台灣大學 A well-known university in Taiwan.

Ou Ye Zi 歐冶子 One of the three most famous sword makers in the Chinese Spring and Autumn Period (722-484 B.C.) and the Warring States Period (403-222 B.C.). The other two well-known sword makers were Gan Jiang and Mo Xie. Ou Ye Zi forged two very famous swords, Ju Que and Zhan Lu.

Pi 劈 Chop or split. One of the basic sword techniques.

Pu Yuan 浦原 A famous sword maker during the Chinese Three Kingdoms Period (221-280 A.D.).

Qi 戚 A common family name in China.

Qi (Chi) 氣 A Chinese term for universal energy. A current popular model is that the Qi circulating in the human body is bioelectric in nature.

Qi Lin Bu 麒麟步 The Unicorn Stance. One of the fundamental stances in northern Chinese martial arts.

Qi Men Jian 戚門劍 The sword techniques and sequences created in Qi's family.

Qi, Ji-Guang 戚繼光 A well known general in the Ming Dynasty (1386-1644 A.D.). Born in 1528 A.D. at Dong Mou Xian in Shandong Province. He studied the martial arts from early childhood onward. His father, Qi, Jing-Tong, was an official in Deng Zhou in charge of guarding the city.

Qi, Jing-Tong 戚景東 Qi, Ji-Guang's father, who was an official in Deng Zhou in charge of guarding the city during Chinese Ming Dynasty (1366-1644 A.D.).

Qigong (Chi Kung) 氣功 The Gongfu of Qi, which means the study of Qi.

Qin (Chin) 擒 Means "to catch" or "to seize."

Qin Na (Chin Na) 擒拿 Literally means "grab control." A component of Chinese martial arts that emphasizes grabbing techniques to control your opponent's joints, in conjunction with attacking certain acupuncture cavities.

Qin Shi 秦始皇 An emperor of the Qin Dynasty (255-206 B.C.).

Qin Yang 沁陽 A county in Henan Province.

Qing Dynasty (1644-1911 A.D.**)** 清朝 One of the dynasties in Chinese history.

Ren 人 Man.

San Cai 三才 Refers to the three powers of heaven, earth, and man in Chinese culture.

San Cai Jian 三才劍 Name of a well-known sequence. It is said that this sequence was created in Xingyiquan style, and is the most well-known matching practice for the sword.

San Guo (220-280 A.D.**)** 三國 The Three Kingdoms Period. One of the periods in Chinese history.

Shang Dynasty (1751-1111 B.C.**)** 商朝 One of the dynasties in Chinese history.

Shaolin 少林 "Young woods." Name of the Shaolin Temple.

Shaolin Temple 少林寺 A monastery located in Henan Province, China. The Shaolin Temple is well known because of its martial arts training.

She-She Jian 蛇舌劍 Snake tongue sword. A type of sword with the blade shaped like a snake's tongue.

Shu 蜀 Sichuan Province is also called Shu.

Si Liu Bu 四六步 The Four-Six Stance. One of the fundamental stances in northern Chinese martial styles.

Sichuan (Shu) 四川省（蜀） A province in western China.

Song Dynasty (960-1280 A.D) 宋朝 One of the dynasties in Chinese history.

Sui and Tang Dynasties (581-907 A.D.**)** 隋、唐 Sui and Tang are two of the dynasties in Chinese history.

Suzhou 蘇州 A city in Jiangsu Province.

Tai Chi Chuan (Taijiquan) 太極拳 A Chinese internal martial style which is based on the theory of Taiji (grand ultimate).

Taiji 太極 Means "grand ultimate." It is this force which generates two poles, Yin and Yang.

Taiji Jian 太極劍 Name of the sword sequence in Taijiquan.

Taijiquan (Tai Chi Chuan) 太極拳 A Chinese internal martial style that is based on the theory of Taiji (grand ultimate).

Taipei 台北 The capital city of Taiwan, located in the north.

Taiwan 台灣 An island to the south-east of mainland China. Also known as "Formosa."

Taiwan University 台灣大學 A well known university located in northern Taiwan.

Taizuquan 太祖拳 A style of Chinese external martial arts.

Tamkang University 淡江大學 A University in northern Taiwan.

Tamkang College Guoshu Club 淡江國術社 A Chinese martial arts club founded by Dr. Yang when he was studying in Tamkang College.

Tian 天 Means "heaven" or "sky."

Tiao 挑　Pluck. One of the basic sword techniques.

Tui Na 推拿　Push and grab. A Chinese Qigong massage technique for healing.

Tuo 托　Bear. One of the basic sword techniques.

Wen Jian 文劍　Scholar sword. The scholar sword, also known as the female sword (Ci Jian), is lighter and shorter than the martial or male sword (Xiong Jian).

Wu 武　Means "martial."

Wu Dai (907-960 A.D.) 五代　The Five Dynasties. A period in Chinese history.

Wu Dan Jian 武當劍　A style of sword techniques and a sequence created at Wudang mountain.

Wu Gou Jian 吳鉤劍　Wu Hooked Sword. This sword was invented during the Wu Dynasty (222-280 A.D.), and is designed for cutting an enemy's limbs, or his horse's legs after blocking their weapons.

Wu Jian 武劍　Martial sword. The martial sword, also known as the male sword (Xiong Jian), is heavier and longer than the scholar or female sword (Ci Jian).

Wu Kang 武康　A county in Zhejiang Province, known for the production of high quality ancient weapons.

Wu Song 武松　A hero in the Chinese Song Dynasty (960-1280 A.D.).

Wushu (Gongfu) 武術(功夫)　Literally, martial technique. It is commonly called Guoshu (i.e., country techniques) in Taiwan or Gongfu in the western society.

Wuyi 武藝　Literally, "martial arts."

Xi 洗　Wash. One of the basic sword techniques.

Xinzhu Xian 新竹縣　Birthplace of Dr. Yang, Jwing-Ming in Taiwan.

Xu Bu (Xuan Ji Bu) 虛步（玄機步）　The False Stance. One of the fundamental stances in northern Chinese martial arts.

Xuan Ji Bu (Xu Bu) 玄機步（虛步）　The False Stance. One of the fundamental stances in northern Chinese martial arts.

Yang Style Taijiquan 楊氏太極拳　A style of Taijiquan created by Yang, Lu-Chan in Qing Dynasty (1644-1911 A.D.).

Yang, Jwing-Ming 楊俊敏　Author of this book.

Yao 搖　Shake. One of the basic sword techniques.

Yuan Dynasty (1206-1368 A.D.) 元朝　One of the dynasties in Chinese history.

Yun 雲　Cloud. One of the basic sword techniques.

Yangzi River 揚子江　Also called Chang Jiang (i.e., long river). One of the two major rivers in China.

Yue Fei 岳飛　A Chinese hero in the Southern Song Dynasty (1127-1279 A.D.). Said to have created Ba Duan Jin, Xingyiquan and Yue's Ying Zhua.

Zhan Guo (403-221 B.C.) 戰國　The Warring States Period. A period in Chinese history.

Zhan Lu 湛盧 One of the two famous swords made by sword maker Ou Ye Zi, during the Chinese Spring and Autumn Period (722-484 B.C.) and the Warring States Period (403-222 B.C.). The other sword was called "Ju Que."

Zhang, Xiang-San 張詳三 A well known Chinese martial artist in Taiwan.

Zhejiang 浙江省 A province of China near the south-east coast.

Zhou Dynasty (1111-221 B.C.**)** 周朝 A dynasty in Chinese history.

Zhuo Lu 涿鹿 Location of an ancient battle between the Emperor Huang Di's forces and his opponent, Chi You.

Zuo Pan Bu 坐盤步 The Crossed Leg Stance. One of the fundamental stances in northern Chinese martial arts.

Index

Books & Videos from YMAA

YMAA Publication Center Books

YMAA Publication Center Videotapes

YMAA Publication Center   楊氏東方文化出版中心

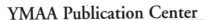

4354 Washington Street Roslindale, MA 02131
1-800-669-8892 • ymaa@aol.com • www.ymaa.com